CHE
AND MEDICINE

CHE
AND MEDICINE

ERNESTO GUEVARA ON THE
SOCIAL ROLE OF DOCTORS

Edited and introduced by
ALEIDA GUEVARA, MD

Centro de Estudios
CHE GUEVARA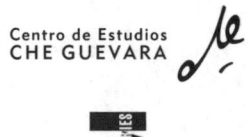

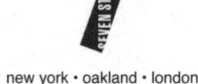

new york • oakland • london

Published by Seven Stories Press on behalf of Ocean Press, Melbourne, Australia, and the Che Guevara Studies Center, Havana. Direct all rights inquiries and permissions questions to rights@sevenstories.com.

ISBN 978-1-64421-425-1 (paperback)
ISBN 978-1-64421-426-8 (ebook)

Also published by Seven Stories Press/Ocean Sur in Spanish as
Che y la medicina, ISBN 978-1-64421-431-2 (paperback);
ISBN 978-1-64421-432-9 (ebook)

Printed in Canada

9 8 7 6 5 4 3 2 1

Contents

ERNESTO CHE GUEVARA
BIOGRAPHICAL NOTE

One of *Time* magazine's "icons of the century," Ernesto Guevara de la Serna was born in Rosario, Argentina, on June 14, 1928. He made several trips around Latin America during and immediately after his studies at medical school in Buenos Aires, including his 1952 journey with Alberto Granado, on the unreliable Norton motorbike described in his travel journal *The Motorcycle Diaries*.

He was already becoming involved in political activity and living in Guatemala when, in 1954, the elected government of Jacobo Árbenz was overthrown in a CIA-organized military operation. Ernesto escaped to Mexico, profoundly radicalized. Following up on a contact made in Guatemala, Guevara sought out the group of Cuban revolutionaries then exiled in Mexico City. In July 1955, he met Fidel Castro and immediately enlisted in the guerrilla expedition to overthrow Cuban dictator Fulgencio Batista. The Cubans nicknamed him "Che," a popular form of address in Argentina.

On November 25, 1956, Che Guevara set sail for Cuba aboard the cabin cruiser *Granma* as the doctor to the guerrilla group that began the revolutionary armed struggle in Cuba's Sierra Maestra mountains. Within several months, he was appointed by Fidel Castro as the first Rebel Army commander, although he continued ministering medically to wounded guerrilla fighters and captured soldiers from Batista's army.

In September 1958, Che Guevara played a decisive role in the military defeat of Batista after he and Camilo Cienfuegos led separate guerrilla columns westward from the Sierra Maestra (later described in his book *Reminiscences of the Cuban Revolutionary War*).

After Batista fled on January 1, 1959, Che Guevara became a key leader of the new revolutionary government, first as head of the Department of Industry of the National Institute of Agrarian Reform; later he became the president of the National Bank. In February 1961 he became minister of industry. He was also a central leader of the political organization that in 1965 became the Communist Party of Cuba.

Apart from these responsibilities, Che Guevara represented the Cuban revolutionary government around the world, heading numerous delegations and speaking at the United Nations and other international forums in Asia, Africa, Latin America and the socialist bloc countries. He earned a reputation as a passionate and articulate spokesperson for the peoples of the Global South, most famously at the conference at Punta del Este in Uruguay, where he denounced US President Kennedy's Alliance for Progress.

As had been his intention since joining the Cuban revolutionary movement, Che Guevara left Cuba in April 1965, initially to lead a Cuban-organized guerrilla mission to support the revolutionary struggle in the Congo, Africa. He returned to Cuba secretly in December 1965 to prepare another Cuban-organized guerrilla force for Bolivia. Arriving in Bolivia in November 1966, Che's plan was to challenge that country's military dictatorship and eventually to instigate a revolutionary movement that would extend throughout the continent of Latin America. Che was wounded and captured by US-trained and run Bolivian counterinsurgency troops on October 8, 1967.

The following day he was murdered and his body hidden. The diary he wrote during this period became known as *The Bolivian Diary*.

Che Guevara's remains were finally discovered in 1997 and returned to Cuba. A memorial was built at Santa Clara in central Cuba, where he had won a major military battle during the revolutionary war.

CHE GUEVARA'S INTERNATIONALIST LEGACY

Ever since the triumph of the Cuban revolution, health care has taken center stage. As early as 1960, a brigade of Cuban doctors was sent to Chile, in the aftermath of a devastating earthquake. Cuba's first official internationalist medical brigade was sent to Algeria in 1963 to provide health care to the population less than a year after that country achieved its independence. Che visited members of that first mission in Algeria a couple of months after their arrival.

Over the past 60 years, Cuban doctors and other medical personnel have offered their services as part of internationalist missions around the world, saving lives and treating millions, many of whom had never previously had access to health care.

In 2005, in response to the destruction caused by Hurricane Katrina in the south of the United States, President Fidel Castro founded the Henry Reeve International Contingent of Doctors Specializing in Disaster Situations and Serious Epidemics. Although the US government refused that offer of solidarity, the brigade has gone on to save lives across the world following earthquakes and other natural disasters, cholera outbreaks, Ebola and, most recently, COVID-19.

Operación Milagro (Operation Miracle), a program launched in 2004 together with the Venezuelan government, has seen millions of people across Latin America and the Caribbean, Africa and Asia receive free medical treatment to restore their eyesight. The often simple procedures were previously inaccessible to those from poor backgrounds.

Cuba's medical expertise has also seen the training of young people from over 70 countries as doctors, through scholarships offered at the Latin American School of Medicine (ELAM), founded in 1999. To counter the constant loss of health workers from the Global South, graduates must commit to return to their home countries on completing their studies to practice where they are most needed.

INTRODUCTION: CHE GUEVARA AND MEDICINE
BY DR. ALEIDA GUEVARA

This book is actually a dream that my mother had for a long time, hoping that I, her eldest daughter, could complete some of my father's work on medicine and the social role of a doctor. But I always explained to her that what my father really wanted to do was to write a very ambitious book (*La función del médico en Latinoamérica* / The Role of the Doctor in Latin America), which he started while he was in Guatemala in 1954. The objective was to show the development of medicine in our continent from pre-Columbian times to colonial and then post-colonial times. Obviously, this would take many years of research and he himself realized that it was a very ambitious project. Nevertheless, he was committed to assisting the new generations to know who we are, where we come from, and to discover our cultural and scientific roots.

When the Spanish conquest occurred, it swept away a whole wealth of medical knowledge that was already being practiced. For example, the Incas performed skull trepanations and, erroneously, many people thought that most of those patients died. But now we know that was not true, many survived. Today, neurosurgeons of Peruvian origin and others in the United States and Canada use the same technique (entrance to the skull through the cleft palate) as the Incas did. Thus, it is extraordinary just how much there is still to be discovered or rediscovered, and how much we must learn about our roots.

There is especially so much ancestral knowledge in our indigenous populations, who are often discriminated against, and marginalized, and yet how useful it would be to improve the lives of our peoples using this knowledge and experience.

This book begins at the University of Buenos Aires, where the young Ernesto Guevara de la Serna studied medicine from 1948 to 1953. Under the tutelage of Dr. Salvador Pisani, Ernesto focused on experimental research on allergies from the start of his degree. We have recovered some of his works that were published at the time.

Here, one can see the development of a young man who has ambitions as a scientist, to be a recognized doctor, perhaps the discoverer of a treatment for leprosy. At the time, lepers were totally marginalized from society.

This book shows a young man who is being shaped by his experiences, who is looking for a way to feel useful as a human being — in this case as a doctor.

His reflections during his travels around Latin America are full of compassion and concern for his fellow human beings.

He arrives in Mexico, and in Mexico he begins to work with Dr. Orlando Torres Salazar Mallén, who was one of the prominent names in Latin American medicine at that time. An outstanding cardiologist, he was also an allergist. A rapport developed with his student, Ernesto Guevara, which later led to a deep friendship.

Later, and in completely different circumstances, Che drafted some guidelines on the treatment of guerrilla fighters who became ill or were wounded in combat in the Sierra Maestra. This experience was reflected in his book *Guerrilla Warfare*, in which he describes what he considers to be the cruelest disease affecting humankind: the poverty to which millions of men and women are subjected, and the indifference of so many others in the face of their suffering.

In compiling this book, I have tried to be faithful to what Che said and wrote and to show how he never stopped being a doctor, even though in the revolutionary war in Cuba he famously had to decide between a box of bullets and a backpack of medicines. Although he opted for the box of bullets, he continued to think like a doctor.

Following the Cuban revolution, Che contributed his ideas and knowledge to the training of a new type of physician, viewing the doctor as an agent of social transformation, with the mission to care for the health of human beings and their environment. He left us some very important speeches about what a revolutionary doctor should be, guidelines for those of us who love our profession and practice it with no profit in mind. As Che said, "the life of a single human being is worth a million times more than all the property of the richest man on earth."

Today, money seems to be everything. People are being bought by money. Nobody claims that money is unnecessary to live. We are all aware that unfortunately "Don Dinero" (Mr. Money) is important, but it cannot be the center of our lives. We have to get beyond that somehow, because medicine is a true vocation. If you devote yourself to being a doctor, it is not to profit from the pain of human beings; it is not to try to get rich from the miseries that thousands and thousands of men and women experience throughout the world.

No, it is to try to improve people's lives. It is to try to make life much better and to make a fairer world for all of us. That is the real role of a physician; because by being so close to human pain, so close to everything that is truly human, we can do a lot for society. That is because we are listened to. If we earn respect as professionals, people will listen to us and that is important.

Che talks about this all the time: how the revolutionary doctor must not just seek to prevent disease. The action of a single, isolated doctor is not enough. We need the action of a whole society. That is why it is essential to have a revolution in order to have revolutionary doctors. And that is one of the things Che showed us throughout his entire life.

Today, Cuba shows the world that we can continue to educate special human beings, despite the criminal US economic blockade we have been subjected to for more than six decades. These Cubans are products of a society that imbues in its children a respect for humanity, men and women who are role models, whose lives encourage and challenge us to continue improving ourselves in order to better serve our people and those of the entire world. In this book, I offer glimpses of a life that is replicated in millions of others today.

Thank you Che, thank you doctor, thank you Dad.

FIRST YEARS

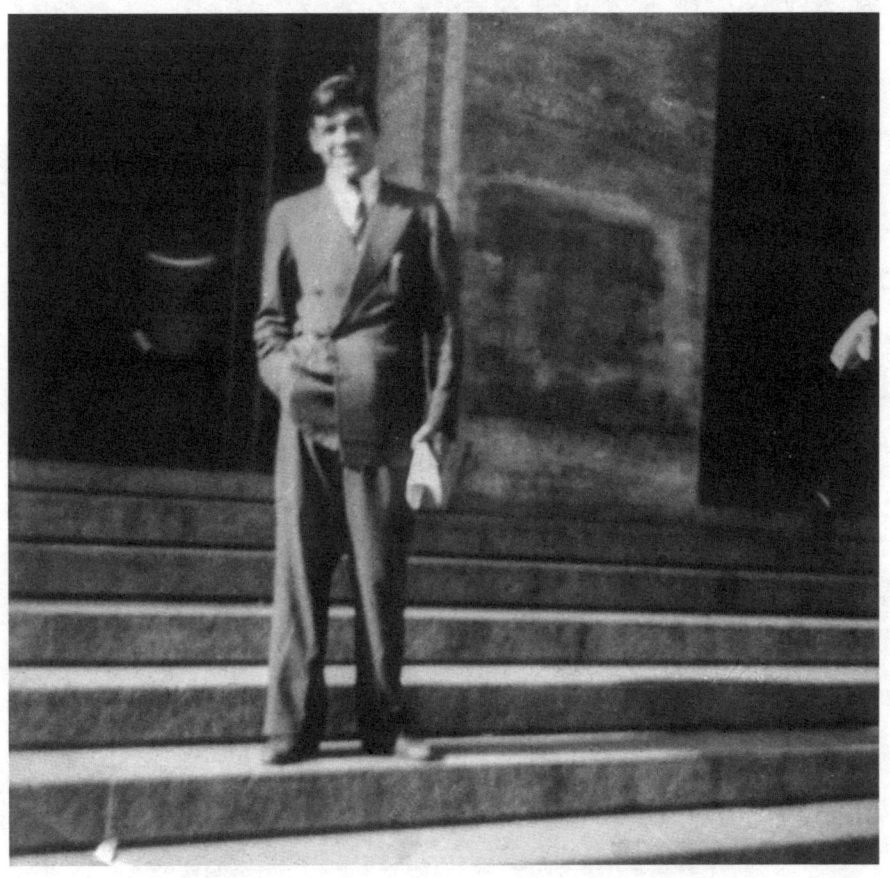

On the steps to the School of Medicine, Buenos Aires, Argentina.

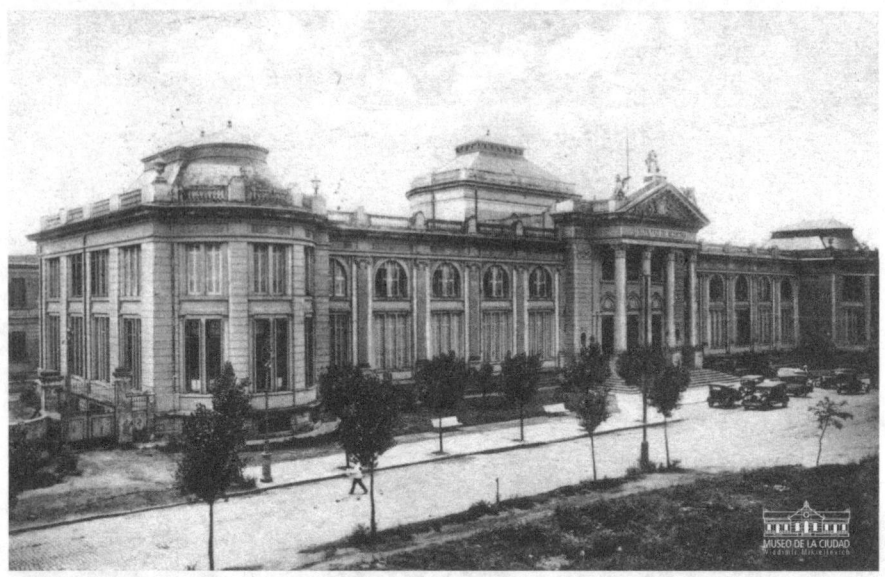

School of Medicine, Santa Fe Street and Francia Avenue, Buenos Aires.

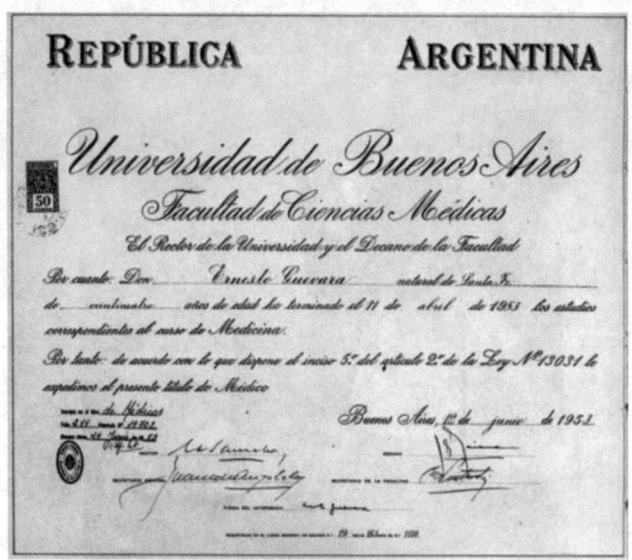

Ernesto Guevara's medical degree certificate.

THE BEGININGS OF A CAREER

In March 1947, Ernesto Guevara's family returned to Buenos Aires from Alta Gracia, Córdoba. His paternal grandmother was seriously ill and young Ernesto would care for her for 17 days, as his father recalls in the book *Mi hijo el Che* (My Son Che). The experience would determine his decision to become a doctor. He enrolled in the School of Medicine that same year.

Ernesto's father describes a very active young man who had to work for a living and refused any financial support from his parents to study medicine. He did many jobs, including working as a nurse for the merchant navy and on oil tankers; later, he was employed as an assistant in the municipal health service and then he worked in Dr. Salvador Pisani's office and laboratory.

He had first met Dr. Pisani as an asthma patient and, according to his father, with the doctor's treatment his condition improved significantly. This inspired Ernesto to specialize in allergies. A close bond was established between the doctor and patient. Later, Ernesto joined a group of young professionals who worked with Dr. Pisani. He undertook various scientific research projects with them, which would later be published in several medical journals.

Ernesto graduated as a doctor on June 12, 1953.

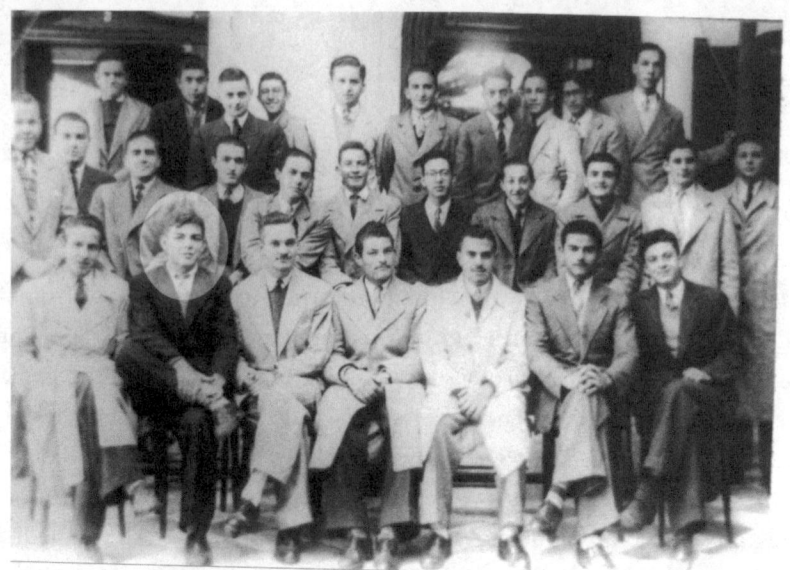

Ernesto (front row) with fellow medical students.

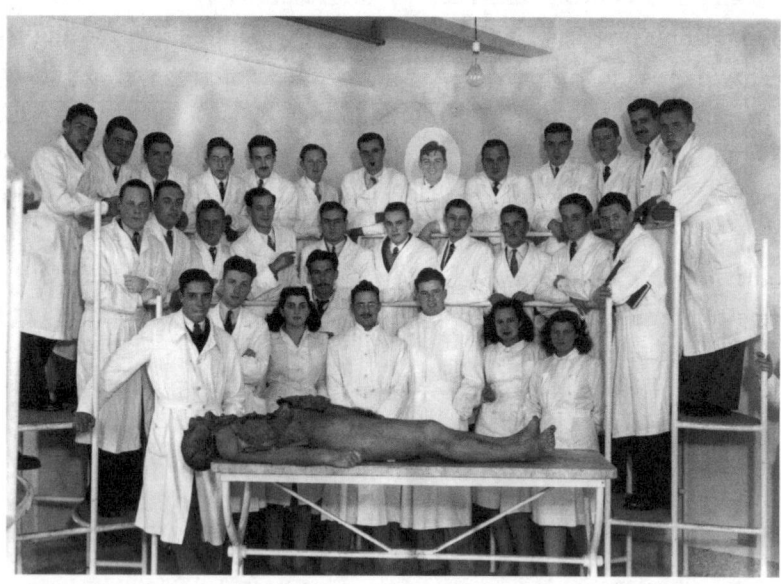

Ernesto (back row) in the School of Medicine anatomy lab alongside his classmates.
Buenos Aires, 1948.

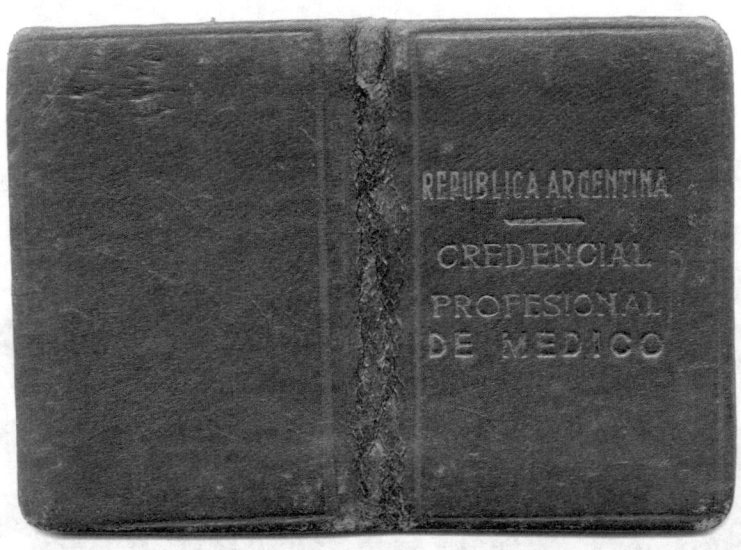

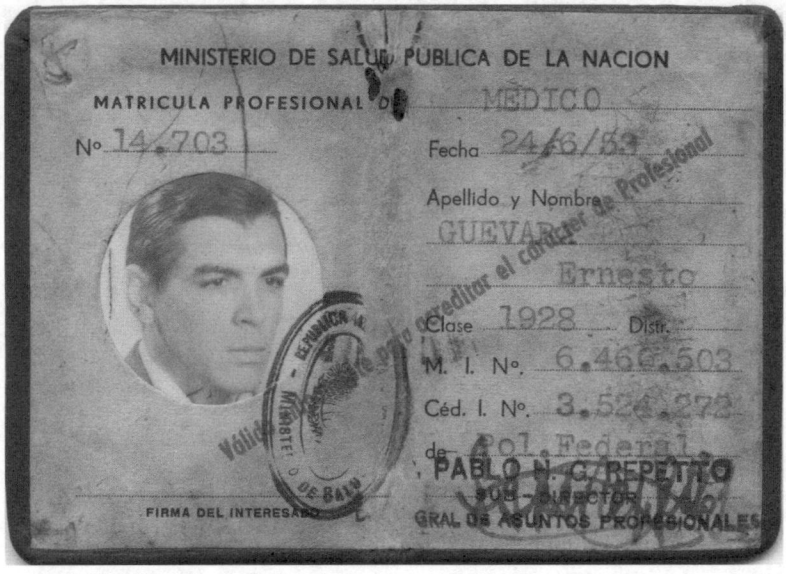

Medical license, issued on June 24, 1953.

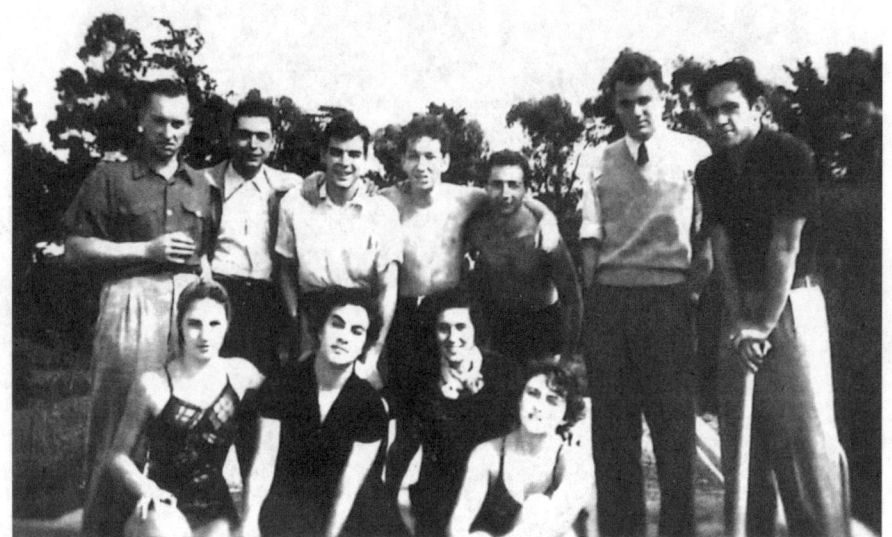

WORKING ALONGSIDE DR. PISANI*

Could you tell us how you came to meet Ernesto Guevara?

I met Ernesto at an allergy institute. I had gone to the institute as I was attempting to see […] I had rhinitis and when I entered the faculty there, the head of the institute, the guy that ran the whole institute side of things, said why don't you come and work with us. Besides learning a lot we won't charge for your studies. So I ended up there. I liked the laboratory and I met other people there who like me had come seeking treatment for an allergy. For example, there was one guy who was asthmatic and always carried a little device which had a rubber bag which he squeezed to release a broncho-dilator called Asmopul. He had been studying at the faculty for longer than I had. We started together with […] the institute director gave us work to do.

And who was that student with asthma?

That student with asthma was called Ernesto, that was all I knew. His name was Ernesto, his last name was Guevara, [...] that was how I met Ernesto in that place, because we were both patients and research assistants in Dr. Salvador Pisani's institute, who I knew was one of the most influential allergists in Argentina at that time.

Could you tell us what your laboratory research consisted of?

Dr. Salvador Pisani had a very original theory. You see with allergies, the mechanism of the allergy is immunological. There is a substance called an antigen, I can explain what that is later if you want, and that forms an anti-

---

*   This is an interview with Dr. Carlos Inglesini, an allergist and Ernesto's compa-
      nion during his student days. As an older man, his memories were not always
      free-flowing. We nevertheless wanted to include excerpts of this interview by
      Argentine journalist Silvia Velarga because there are so few reminiscences about
      Ernesto in those years.

body. This is an antibody that is not a protective antibody; on the contrary, it is an antibody that produces disease. The protective antibody is immunoglobulin G and that which produces an allergy is immunoglobulin E.

Pisani said that in order for there to be a reaction to pollen, there had to be some sort of sensitivity. There had to be a substance that produced an antibody that acted as if it were produced by the pollen. He called this antigenic coincidence. That is to say, that a substance produces an antibody and eventually other substances that have nothing to do with this, for example, as I explained before, a pollen, a grass, this pollen could react with a food like egg, chocolate, pork, for example. So there has to be an already existing antibody, the antibody which is an immunoglobulin E, which was already formed so that when the coincidental substance appears, which for example is the pollen, it binds to the antibody not produced by the pollen itself, which was produced by another element, for example the food I mentioned. This coincidence between the antibody produced by a food and that produced by a pollen is what causes the symptoms. That is the antigenic coincidence and it was the topic that Salvador assigned us. He gave it to Ernesto to work on and Ernesto told me: "Look, we're going to work on this because it's very important."

Doctor, do you remember when Che, (Ernesto), left on a motorcycle to travel around Latin America? Did he say goodbye to you all before setting off?

On one of Ernesto's trips, I think it was the first trip… he said goodbye as he left for Chile. He set off from the laboratory in Palermo and those of us who were working there came out onto the street to wave him off. He was traveling with a friend, I don't know if it was [Alberto] Granado or his other friend, I can't remember. But I remember that he was carrying two suitcases, a small case and a bigger one. They took books and clothes. In the big case they took books and in the small case clothes. And there was another detail, I have no idea why I remember this, but Ernesto was wearing a light blue shirt and gray pants.

Do you remember what Pisani said to him when they left on the motorcycle?

Well, Pisani also noticed that and said: "What! You're taking more books than clothes, Ernesto!" and he laughed.

And did you see him when he returned from that trip?

We saw him... he told us about his trip... Ernesto came back and he told us that he had spent a month living with — I don't know if they were indigenous people or some community of that kind — who, he said, were utterly exploited and treated like animals... He was very concerned about those people and he always said that something had to be done for them, that they couldn't continue to live like that. That is, that we had to do something, somehow, to stop people from being treated like that.

When he returned from that trip, he still had some subjects to pass in order to graduate. There are several final subjects in medicine, seven or eight different subjects, I can't remember. But they are short courses as they are specialties. Ernesto took all those exams and once he had finished, the entire laboratory staff honored him with a barbecue at the country house of the laboratory patron, Mr. Benjamín Duó.

And then he set off on his second trip.

We didn't see him again after he left for his second trip. I heard nothing more from him and we didn't know what was happening in Cuba. But when we heard that the Cuban revolution had triumphed and that Commander Fidel Castro had reached Havana and that his second-in-command was the Argentine Che Guevara I said: "Hey! It's Ernesto!"

And how do you think that Ernesto, with his asthma, was able to be a guerrilla and endure that struggle in such a humid climate?

It's a tough question to answer. What I can say is that asthma is obviously a very serious disability, making it very hard to undertake great physical exertion. But it appears that strength of will is more important than bronchial physiology.

Dr. SALVADOR PISANI y Sres. J. M. y M. POIRON,
E. GUEVARA y H. SCHERB

PRODUCCION EXPERIMENTAL DE DISPOSICION ALERGICA HEREDADA EN EL COBAYO

Apartado de la Revista
LA SEMANA MEDICA
Tomo 100 - N° 17 - Abril 24 de 1952

BUENOS AIRES
1952

Section of the magazine *La semana médica*, featuring an article coauthored by Ernesto Guevara, April 1952.

HISTAMINASA EN SUERO DE MUJERES ALERGICAS
EN EL CURSO DEL EMBARAZO

Dr. Salvador Pisani, Sra. Amelia María G. M. de Duhau y Sr. J. M. Poirón

Año LXIV – N⁰ 3327 – Tomo 111 – N⁰ 7 – Agosto 15 de 1957

DOSAJE DE HISTAMINASA EN ORGANOS HUMANOS

Dres. Salvador Pisani, Ernesto Guevara, W. Sánchez de la Vega,
Sr. J. M. Poirón y Srta. Liria Bocciolesi

Año LXIV – N⁰ 3338 – Tomo 111 – N⁰ 18 – Octubre 31 de 1957

DOSAJE DE HISTAMINASA EN ORGANOS DE ANIMALES

Dres. Salvador Pisani, W. Sánchez de la Vega, Sr. Juan M. Poirón
y Srta. Liria Bocciolesi

Año LXIV – N⁰ 3329 – Tomo 111 – N⁰ 9 – Agosto 29 de 1957

HISTAMINASA EN PLACENTA HUMANA Y MANIFES-
TACIONES ALERGICAS PRECOCES EN EL HIJO

Dres. Salvador Pisani, Manuel Asrilant, Sra. A. M. G. M. de Duhau,
Sr. J. M. Poirón y Srta. Liria Bocciolesi

Año LXIV – N⁰ 3337 – Tomo 111 – N⁰ 17 – Octubre 24 de 1957

MANIFESTACIONES ALERGICAS MATERNAS EN EL
CURSO DEL EMBARAZO Y MANIFESTACIONES
ALERGICAS PRECOCES EN EL HIJO

Dres. Salvador Pisani, W. Sánchez de la Vega y Sr. J. M. Poirón

Año LXIV – N⁰ 3335 – Tomo 111 – N⁰ 15 – Octubre 10 de 1957

□

Apartados de la revista, LA SEMANA MÉDICA

□

BUENOS AIRES
1957

Section of the magazine *La semana médica*, featuring an article coauthored
by Ernesto Guevara, 1957.

DOSAJE DE HISTAMINASA EN ORGANOS HUMANOS

POR LOS DOCTORES

SALVADOR PISANI, ERNESTO GUEVARA, W. SÁNCHEZ DE LA VEGA,
Sr. J. M. POIRON y Srta. LIRIA BOCCIOLESI

CONOCEMOS en forma más o menos aproximada el papel de la histamina o sustancias "H" en el desencadenamiento de las reacciones anafilácticas y de las reacciones alérgicas.

Como la sustancia específicamente destructora de la histamina en el organismo es la histaminasa, quisimos determinar la tasa de esta sustancia en algunos órganos humanos. Sabemos que la histaminasa es una enzima que posee, al parecer, una constitución proteica y se encuentra comprendida dentro de la fracción globulínica de las proteínas. Dicha enzima es difícilmente dosable en la sangre humana, salvo en mujeres portadoras de embarazo, en las que a partir del tercer mes del mismo empieza a aparecer en sangre y se eleva en forma paulatina hasta el sexto mes en que alcanza un nivel tope en el que se mantiene hasta el final del embarazo Estos trabajos serán motivo de otra comunicación.

La técnica que usamos para la determinación de la tasa de histaminasa es la siguiente:

Se toman 4 g de órgano, se desintegran y se suspenden en este 10 cm³ de Buffer, durante 24 horas en heladera. A continuación se centrifuga y con el líquido sobrenadante se preparan dos muestras; la primera con 2 cm³ y la segunda con 5 cm³. Se completan ambas a 9 cm³ con solución fisiológica a pH 7. Se agrega luego 1 cm³ de diclorhidrato de histamina 1:100.000 en solución fisiológica. Se prepara una solución testigo que contenga 9 cm³ de solución fisiológica a pH 7 y 1 cm³ de histamina 1:100.000. Todas estas muestras se mantienen a 37º durante 1 hora en la estufa. Terminada la incubación se congelan rápidamente y se mantienen a menos 20º hasta el momento de su medición.

Los órganos estudiados fueron hígado, intestino, pulmón y riñón. Como considerábamos que pudiera haber diferencia en el nivel histaminolítico de los órganos en individuos adultos y niños, tomamos a ambos por separado, pero como veremos ulteriormente, no ha habido una diferencia apreciable entre los niveles observados en unos y otros.

Se estudiaron los órganos de 34 niños y 92 adultos. Se consideró la mayor cantidad de factores que nos parecieron capaces de alterar el nivel histaminolítico de los órganos.

Los niños estudiados tenían hasta 12 años de edad y se trató de establecer relaciones entre la tasa de histaminasa y los siguientes factores: se tomaron en cuenta las diversas edades; hasta 1 mes, 3 meses, 1 año, y de 1 a 12 años, y no se encontró ninguna relación con estos factores. Lo mismo puede decirse con respecto al sexo. Se trató de determinar la importancia del tiempo transcurrido entre el día de la muerte, día de la autopsia y día en que se realizó la investigación. Se trató de establecer relación con síntomas o signos observados en el enfermo, tales como vómitos, diarreas, obnubilación, deshidratación, disnea, convulsiones, ictericia, fiebre y en este último caso se consideraron los días en que se mantuvo el proceso febril; no encontrándose relación con ninguno de los factores anotados.

Los diagnósticos clínicos fueron los siguientes: toxicosis, osteomielitis, sarampión y coqueluche. La medicación empleada en el curso de la enfermedad que los llevó a la muerte fueron las siguientes: antibióticos (todos), digital, insulina, éter, vitaminas, nicotibina, analépticos, hormonas adrenales, antiespasmódicos, sedantes (barbitúricos, bromuros), ginergeno, morfina, antihistamínicos, sulfas, diuréticos, adrenalina, transfusiones, foliculina, progesterona, luteína, oxígeno, prostigmín, epamín, extracto hepático, hialuronidasa, testovirón, antitérmicos (aspirina, criogenina, fenacetina), piramidón y cafeína.

Las lesiones anátomopatológicas encon-

Section of the magazine *La semana médica,* featuring an article coauthored by Ernesto Guevara, 1957.

TRANSMISION PASIVA DE LA SENSIBILIDAD PARA ANTIGENO DE TENIA SAGINATA

DOS CASOS

POR

Dr. Salvador Pisani,
Sr. J. M. Poirón,
Sra. M. Pisani de Poirón,
Dr. Ernesto Guevara

LEÍDO EN LA SOCIEDAD ARGENTINA DE ALERGIA
el 3 de diciembre de 1953

Apartado de la Revista
A L E R G I A
Vol. I – Noviembre de 1953 – Nº 2

Section of the magazine *La semana médica*, featuring an article coauthored by Ernesto Guevara, 1957.

TRANSMISION PASIVA DE LA SENSIBILIDAD PARA ANTIGENO DE TENIA SAGINATA

DOS CASOS

Dr. Salvador Pisani, Sr. J. M. Poirón, señora M. Pisani de Poirón, Dr. Ernesto Guevara.

Vamos a describir dos casos de enfermos alérgicos que sufrían una parasitación por *Tenia Saginata*, los dos resultan de verdadero interés, porque en ambos el parásito actuaba como agente desencadenante de la manifestación alérgica y como se verá más adelante existía una "real" sensibilización clínica para el mismo y en fin se demostró la presencia de anticuerpos circulantes en los enfermos parasitados por la prueba de transmisión pasiva con la técnica de Prausnitz-Küstner.

CASO Núm. 1: P. S., Sexo: Femenino. Edad: 19 años. Fecha de ingreso: 12 VIII/'49.

Antecedentes hereditarios y familiares: sin importancia.

Antecedentes personales: difteria a los 8 años, tratada con suero. Enfermedad actual: primera crisis de asma a los 7 años y desde entonces continuaron ininterrumpidamente hasta los 14 años en que entró en un período de calma espontáneo, en febrero de 1949, nueva crisis de asma y rinitis vasomotora que continúa hasta la fecha.

Estado actual: Pulmones, sibilancias en ambos campos. Corazón, normal. Hígado, 1 través del reborde. Resto, sin interés.

Análisis clínicos: Kahn estandard y presuntiva, negativa, Eritrosedimentación, 1ra. 14, 2da. 35. Orina normal. Materia fecal, *ameba histolítica* forma vegetativa. *Blastocystis hominis*. Esputo, flora banal.

INVESTIGACION ALERGICA

Pólenes: negativos. Inhalantes: sensibilización moderada a pluma de gallina, pavo, pato y ganso. Estopa, esparto, kapock (paina), crin, manta de algodón (guata), lana y detritus vegetales; y fuerte a polvo

— 3 —

Section of the magazine *La semana médica,* featuring an article coauthored by Ernesto Guevara, 1957.

FIRST TRIP AROUND LATIN AMERICA

The person who wrote these notes passed away the moment his feet touched Argentine soil again. The person who reorganizes and polishes them, me, is no longer, at least I am not the person I once was. All this wandering around "Our America with a capital A" has changed me more than I thought.

So writes Che in the introduction to his ***The Motorcycle Diaries: Notes on a Latin American Journey*,** **from which we take several excerpts related to his early experiences as a doctor.**

"La Gioconda's smile"

[…] We tried to contact the doctors from Petrohué, but being back at work with no time to spare, they never agreed to meet us formally. At least we knew more or less where they were. In the afternoon we went our separate ways: while Alberto followed up the doctors, I went to see an old woman with asthma, a client at La Gioconda. The poor thing was in a pitiful state, breathing the acrid smell of concentrated sweat and dirty feet that filled her room, mixed with the dust from a couple of armchairs, the only luxury items in her house. On top of her asthma, she had a heart condition. It is at times like this, when a doctor is conscious of his complete powerlessness, that he longs for change: a change to prevent the injustice of a system in which only a month ago this poor woman was still earning her living as a waitress, wheezing and panting but facing life with dignity. In circumstances like this, individuals in poor families who can't pay their way become surrounded by an atmosphere of barely disguised acrimony; they stop being father, mother, sister or brother and become a purely negative factor in the struggle for life and, consequently, a source of bitterness for the healthy members of the community who resent their illness as if it were a personal insult to those who have to support them. It is there, in the final moments, for people whose

farthest horizon has always been tomorrow, that one comprehends the profound tragedy circumscribing the life of the proletariat the world over. In
those dying eyes there is a submissive appeal for forgiveness and also, often,
a desperate plea for consolation which is lost to the void, just as their body
will soon be lost in the magnitude of the mystery surrounding us. How long
this present order, based on an absurd idea of caste, will last is not within my
means to answer, but it's time that those who govern spent less time publici-
zing their own virtues and more money, much more money, funding socially
useful works.

There isn't much I can do for the sick woman. I simply advise her to
improve her diet and prescribe a diuretic and some asthma pills. I have a few
Dramamine tablets left and I give them to her. When I leave, I am followed
by the fawning words of the old woman and the family's indifferent gaze.

Alberto had tracked down the doctors. At nine the following morning
we had to be at the hospital. *(From* **The Motorcycle Diaries,** *"La Gioconda's
Smile.")*

Chile, a vision from afar

Beginning with our area of expertise, medicine: the panorama of health
care in Chile leaves a lot to be desired (although I realized later it was by far
superior to that in other countries I got to know). Free, public hospitals are
extremely rare and even in those, posters announcing the following appear:
"Why do you complain about your treatment if you are not contributing to
the maintenance of this hospital?" Generally speaking, medical attention in
the north is free, but hospital accommodation has to be paid for, and prices
range from petty sums to virtual monuments to legalized theft. Sick or inju-
red workers at the Chuquicamata mine receive medical attention and hospital treatment for five Chilean *escudos* a day, but someone not working at
the mine would pay between 300 and 500 *escudos* a day. Hospitals have no
money and they lack medicine and adequate facilities. We have seen filthy
operating rooms with pitiful lighting, not just in small towns but even in
Valparaíso. There aren't enough surgical instruments. The bathrooms are
dirty. Awareness of hygiene is poor. It's a Chilean custom (afterwards I saw
it across practically all of South America) not to throw used toilet paper in
the toilet but on to the floor or in the boxes provided.

[…]

Chile as a nation offers economic promise to any person disposed to work for it, so long as they don't belong to the proletariat: that is, anyone who has a certain dose of education and technical knowledge. The land has the capacity to sustain enough livestock (especially sheep) and cereals to provide for its population. There are the necessary mineral resources to transform it into a powerful industrial country: iron, copper, coal, tin, gold, silver, manganese and nitrates. The biggest effort Chile should make is to shake its uncomfortable Yankee friend from its back, a task that for the moment at least is Herculean, given the quantity of dollars the United States has invested and the ease with which it flexes its economic muscle whenever its interests appear threatened. *((From* **The Motorcycle Diaries,** *"Chile, A Vision From Afar.")*

The Huambo Leper Colony, Peru

The following morning we went to pay a visit to the patients in the little hospital. The people who are in charge do a great job, even if it goes unnoticed. The general state of the place is disastrous; two-thirds of a small area — the size of less than half a block — is designated as a "sick zone," and in it the entire lives of the 31 condemned take place. They pass the time watching indifferently for death to arrive (at least that's what I think). Sanitary conditions are appalling, and though this might cause no adverse effects on the Indians from the mountains, people coming from other parts, even if only slightly more educated, find it enormously distressing. The thought of having to spend their whole lives between four adobe walls, surrounded by people speaking another language, with only four orderlies who make just short visits each day, causes nervous breakdowns.

We went into a room with a straw roof, its ceiling slatted with cane and an earth floor where a white girl was reading *Cousin Basilio* by Queirós. No sooner had we begun to talk when the girl broke down, crying inconsolably, describing her life as a "calvary," a living hell. The poor girl, from the Amazonian regions, had gone to Cuzco where they gave her the bad news, and said they would send her to a much better place to be cured. The hospital in Cuzco, by no means perfect, did have a certain level of comfort. I believe her expression, the word calvary, was the only just expression for the girl's situation. The only acceptable thing in this hospital was the drug treatment, the rest could have been borne only by the suffering, fatalistic spirit of the Peruvian mountain Indians.

The imbecility of the neighboring locals only heightened the isolation of both patients and medical staff. One of them told us that the head surgeon at the clinic needed to perform a more or less serious operation, impossible at any rate to execute on a kitchen table and lacking the appropriate surgical equipment. So he asked for a place, even if it was the morgue, in a nearby hospital at Andahuaylas. The answer was negative, and the patient died without treatment. *(From* **The Motorcycle Diaries,** *"Huambo.")*

Experiencing first-hand the lives of those with leprosy

The afternoon we dedicated to becoming familiar with the leprosy hospital [Hospital de Guía] with a guided tour by Dr. Molina, who, as well as being a good leprologist, is apparently an excellent thoracic surgeon. As was our custom by then, we went to eat at Dr. Pesce's.

[…]

We spent the afternoon exploring the laboratory, which didn't have much worth envying and, in fact, left a lot to be desired. The bibliographic records, however, were formidable in their clarity and method of organization and also in their comprehensive detail. At night, of course, we were off to Dr. Pesce's for dinner, and as always he proved his skill in animated conversation.

[…]

In spite of its simplicity, one of the things which left a very strong impression on us in Lima was the way the hospital patients farewelled us. They had all chipped in one hundred and a half soles, which they gave to us along with an effusive letter. Afterwards some of them came to say goodbye to us personally and in more than one case tears were shed as they thanked us for the little bit of life we'd given them. We shook their hands, accepted their gifts, and sat with them listening to football on the radio. If there's anything that will make us seriously dedicate ourselves to leprosy, it will be the affection shown to us by all the sick we've met along the way. *(From* **The Motorcycle Diaries,** *"The City of the Viceroys.")*

[Ernesto and Alberto finally arrive at the San Pablo Leprosy Colony]

On Monday we sent a good proportion of our clothes to be washed, then went to the colony to visit the patients' compound. There are 600 sick people living independently in typical jungle huts, doing whatever they choose, looking after themselves, in an organization which has developed a rhythm and style of its own. There is a local official, a judge, a policeman, etc. The respect Dr. Bresciani commands is considerable and he clearly coordinates the whole colony, both protecting and sorting out disputes that arise between the different groups.

On Tuesday we visited the colony again, joining Dr. Bresciani as he made his rounds, examining the patients' nervous systems. He is preparing a detailed study of nervous forms of leprosy based on 400 cases. It really is very interesting work because many of the cases of leprosy in this region attack the nervous system. Actually, I didn't see a single patient who wasn't presenting such symptoms. Bresciani told us that Dr. Souza Lima was interested in early signs of nervous disorder among the children living in the colony.

We went to the part of the colony reserved for the healthy, where 70 or so people live. It is lacking basic amenities that are supposedly being installed, like electricity during the day, a refrigerator and even a laboratory. They are in need of a good microscope, a microtome, a technician — at the moment this post is occupied by Mother Margarita, nice but not very knowledgeable — and they need a surgeon to operate on nerves, eyes, etc. An interesting thing is that aside from the widespread neurological problems, there are very few blind people, perhaps leading to the conclusion that [indecipherable word] has something to do with it, seeing that most receive no treatment at all. *(From* **The Motorcycle Diaries,** *"The San Pablo Leper Colony.")*

Saint Guevara's Day

Tuesday morning, with Alberto fully recovered, we went to the compound where Dr. Montoya had operated on the ulna in a leprous nervous system with apparently brilliant results, although the technique left much to be desired.

[...]

That night an assembly of the colony's patients gave us a farewell serenade, with lots of local songs sung by a blind man. The orchestra was made up of a flute player, a guitarist and an accordion player with almost no fingers, and a "healthy" contingent helping out with a saxophone, a guitar and some percussion. After that came the time for speeches, in which four patients spoke as well as they could, a little awkwardly. One of them froze, unable to go on, until out of desperation he shouted, "Three cheers for the doctors!" Afterwards, Alberto thanked them warmly for their welcome, saying that Peru's natural beauty could not compare with the emotional beauty of this moment, that he had been deeply touched, that he could say no more except… and here he extended his arms with Perón-like gesture and intonation, "I want to give my thanks to all of you." *(From* **The Motorcycle Diaries,** *"Saint Guevara's Day.")*

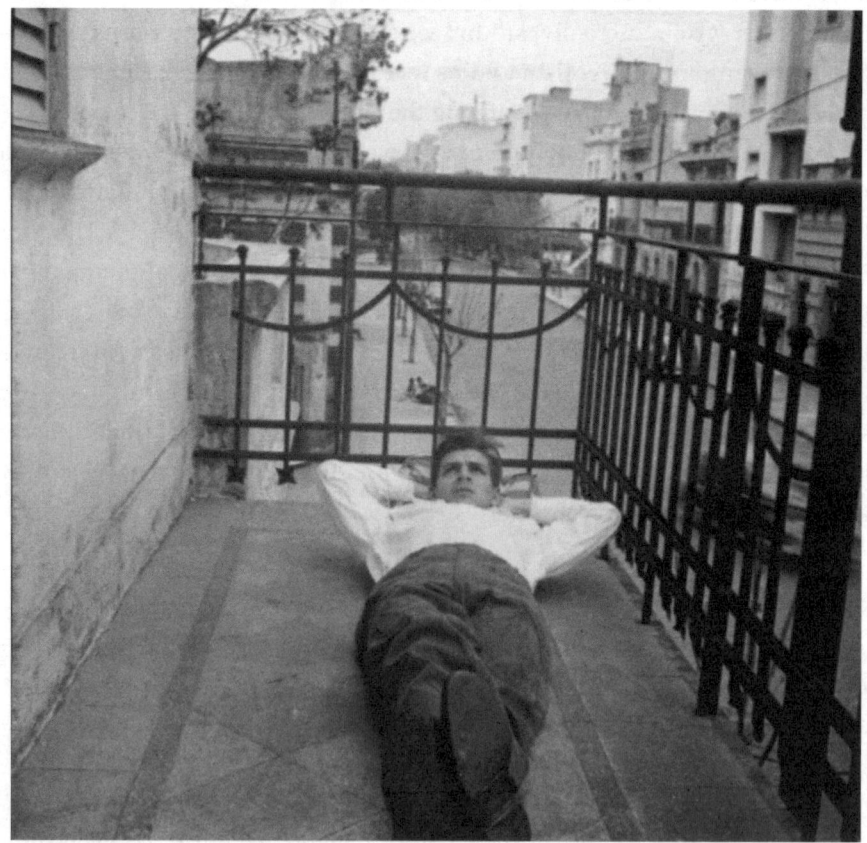

Ernesto in Buenos Aires in 1951 before starting his first trip around Latin America.

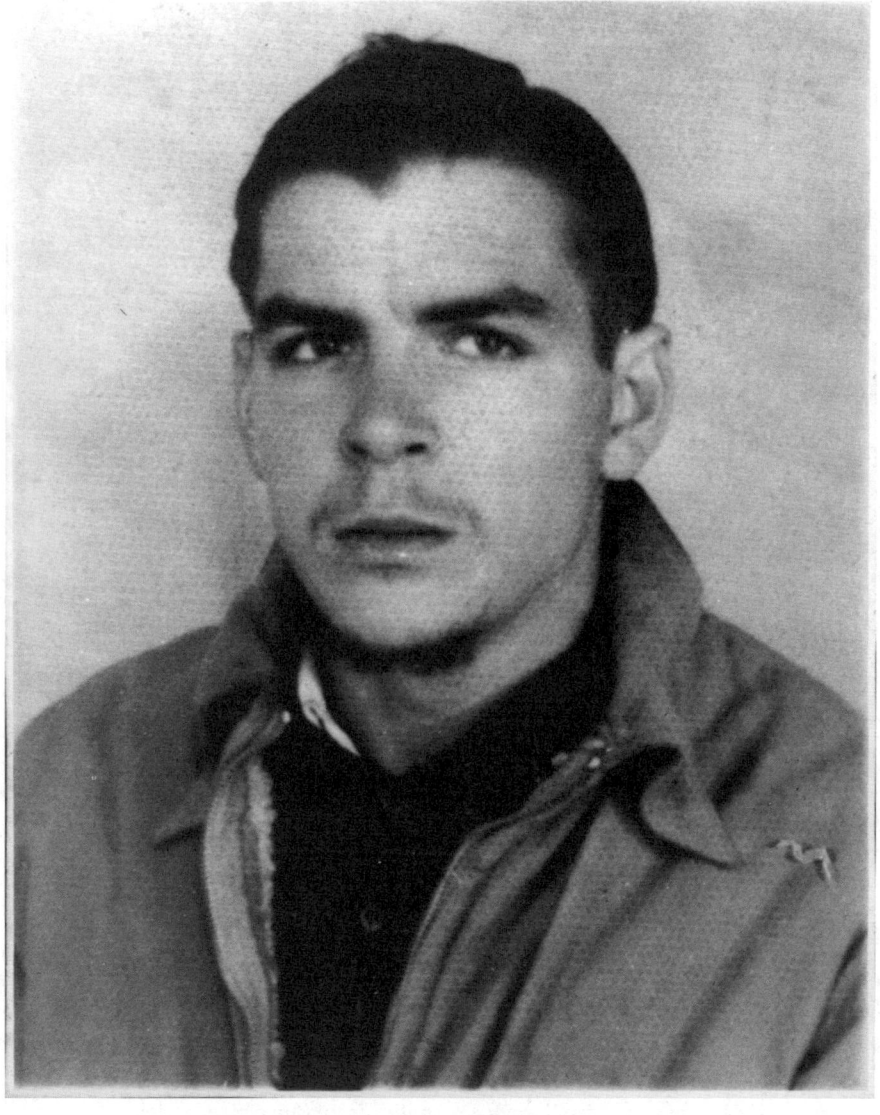

MINISTERIO DE INDUSTRIA Y COMERCIO
DE LA NACION

DIRECCION DE VINOS

LA SONRISA DE LA GIOCONDA

Esta era una nueva parte de la aventura;estábamos acostumbrados a llamar
la atención de los ociosos con nuestros originales atuendos y la pro-
saica figura de la poderosa II xxx cuyo asmático resoplido llenaba de
compasión a nuestros huéspedes,pero,hasta cierto punto,éramos los caba-
lleros del camino. Pertenecíamos a la rancia aristocracia "vaguería" y
traía mos la tarjeta de presentación de nuestros títulos que impresiona
ban inmejorablemente. Ahora no,ya no éramos más que dos linyeras con el
"mono" a cuestas y con toda la mugre del camino condensada en los mame-
lucos,resabio de nuestra aristocrática condición pasada. El conductor
del camión nos había dejado en la parte alta de la ciudad,a la entrada,
y nosotros,con paso cansino,arrastrábamos nuestros bultos calle abajo
seguidas por la mirada divertida e indiferente de los xxxxxxx transeun
tes. El puerto mostraba a lo lejos su tentador brillo de barcos mientras
el mar,negro y cordial,nos llamaba a gritos con su olor gris que dilata
ba nuestras fosas nasales. Compramos pan-el mismo pan que tan caro nos
parecía en ese momento y encontraríamos tan barato al llegar a los lejos
aún-y seguimos calle abajo. Alberto mostraba su cansancio yaye,sin mos-
trarlo,lo tenía tan positivamente instalado como el suyo,de modo que al
llegar a una playa para caminnes y automoviles a saltamos al encargado
con nuestras caras de tragedia,contando en un florido lenguaje los pade
cimientos soportados en la ruda caminata desde Santiago. El viejo nos
cedió un lugar para xxxx dormir,sobre unas ta blas,en comunidad con algunos
parásito de esos xxx cuyo nombre acaba en Hominis,pero bajo techo y ata
camos al sueño con resolución. Sin embargo,nuestra llegada había impre-
sionado los oídos de un compatriota instalado en la fonda adjunta,el que
se apresuró a llamarnos para homenajearnos. Conocer en Chile significa
convidar y ninguno de los dos estaba en condiciones de rechazar el maná
Nuestro paisano demostraba estar profundamente compenetrado con el es-
píritu de la tierra hermana y consecuentemente,tenía una curda de órdago
Hacía tanto tiempo que no comía pescado,y el vino estaba tan rico y el
hombre era tan obsequioso;bueno,comimos bien, y nos invitó a su casa pa
ra el día siguiente.
Temprano la Gioconda abrió sus puertas y sebamos nuestros mates cha rla
lando con el dueño que estaba muy interesado en nuestro viaje. Enseguida,a conocer la ciudad. Valparaíso es muy pintoresca,edificada sobre la
playa que da a la bahía,al crecer,ha ido trepando los cerros que mueren
en el mar. Su extraña arquitectura de zinc,escalonada en gradas que se
unen si por serpenteantes escaleras o por funiculares,ve realzada
su belleza de museo de manicomio por el contraste que forman los diver-
sos coloridos de las casas que se mezclan con el azul plomizo de la bahía. Con paciencia de disectores husmeamos en las suciedades sucias y
en los huecos,charlamos con los mendigos que pululan;auscultamos el fon
do de la ciudad,las miasmas xxx que nos atraen. Nuestras narices dis-
tendidas ca ptan la miseria con fervor sádico.
Visitamos los barcos en el muelle paraver si alguno sale hacia la isla
de Pascua pero las noticias son desalentadoras,ya que hasta dentro de 6
meses no sale ningún buque en esa dirección. Recogimos vagos datos de
unos aviones que hacían vuelos una vez por mes.
La isla de Pascua! La imaginación detiene su vuelo ascendente y queda
dando vueltas en torno a ella: "allí tener un"novio" blanco es un honor
para ellas". "Allí,trabajar,que esperanza,las mujeres hacentodo,uno come
duerme y las tiene contentas.". Ese lugar maravilloso donde el clima es
ideal,las mujeres ideales,la comida ideal,el trabajo ideal(en su beatí-
fica inexistencia). Que importa quedarse un año allí,que importa estudios,sueldos,familia,etc. Desde un escaparate una enorme langosta de mar
nos guiña un ojo,y desde las cuatro lechugas que le sirven de lecho nos
dice con todo su cuerpo:soy de la isla de Pascua;allí dónde está el cli
ma ideal,las mujeres ideales...

Facsimiles of "La Gioconda's Smile," from Che's manuscript
of *The Motorcycle Diaries*.

MINISTERIO DE INDUSTRIA Y COMERCIO
DE LA NACION

DIRECCION DE VINOS

En la puerta de "la Gioconda" esperábamos pacientemente al compatriota que no daba señales de vida,cuando el dueño se comidió a hacernos entrar pa ra que no nos diera el sol y acto seguido nos convidó con una de sus magní ficos almuerzos a base de pescado frito y sopa de agua. De nuestro coterráneo no tuvimos má a noticias en toda nuestra estadía en Valparaíso,pero nos hi cimos íntimos del dueño del boliche. Este era un tipo extraño,indolente y lleno de una caridad enorme para cuanto bicho viviente fuera de lo normal x se acercara hasta su puerta,cobraba,sin embargo, a precio de oro a los clien tes normales,las cuatro perquerías que despachaba en su negocio. En los días que nos quedamos allí no pagamos un centavo y nos llenó de atenciones;hoy por ti,mañana por mi... era su dicho preferido,lo que no indicaría gran ori ginalidad pero era muy efectivo.

Tratábamos de establecer contacto directo con los médicos de Petrohué pe ro estos vueltos a sus quehaceres y sin tiempo para perder,nunca se avenían a una entrevista formal,sin embargo ya los habíamos localizado más o menos bien y esa tarde nos dividimos,mientras Alberto les seguía los pasos yo me fuí a ver una vieja asmática que era clienta dela Gioconda. La pobre daba lástima,se respiraba en su pieza ese olor acre de sudor concentrado y patas sucias,mezclado al polvo de unos sillones,unica paquetería de la casa. Suma ba a su estado asmático una regular descompensación cardíaca. Frente a estos casos es cuando el médico consciente de su total inferioridad frente al me dio,desea un cambio de cosas salga que suprima la injusticia que supone el que la pobre vieja hubiera estado sirviendo hasta hacía un mes para ganarse el sustente,hipando y penando pero manteniendo frente a la vida una actitud erecta. Es q ue la adaptación al medio hace que en las familias pobres el miembro de ellas incapacitado para ganarse el sustente se vea rodeado de un atmósfera de acritud apenas disimulada;en ese momento se deja de ser padre madre o hermano para convertirse en un factor negativo en la lucha por la vida y como tal,objeto del rencor de la comunidad sana que se hecha en cara su enfermedad como si fuera un insulto personal a los sanos que deben mante nerlos. Allí,en estos últimos momentos de gente cuyo horizonte más lejano fué siempre el día de mañana,es donde se capta la profunda tragedia que en cierra la vida del proletariado de todo el mundo;hay en esos ojos moribundo un sumiso o pedido de disculpas y tambien,muchas veces,un desesperado pedido de consuelo que se pierde en el vacío,como se perderá pronto su cuerpo en la magnitud del misterio que nos rodea. Hasta cuando seguirá este orden de cosas basado en un absurdo sentido de casta es algo que no está en mi contestar pero es hora de que los gobernantes dediquen menos tiempo a la propaganda de sus bondades como régimen y más dinero,muchísimo más dinero,a solventar obras de utilidad social. Mucho no puedo hacer por la enferma: simplemente le doy un régimen aproximado de comidas y le recete un diurético y unos pol vos antiasmáticos. Me quedan unas pastillas de dramamina y se las regale. Cuando salgo,me siguen las palabras salameras de la vieja y las miradas indi ferentes de los familiares.

Alberto ya cazó al médico: al día siguiente a las 9 de la mañana hay que estar en el hospital. En el cuartucho que sirve de cocina,comedor,lavadero, comedor y miadero de perros y gatos,hay una reunión heterogenea. El dueño, con su filosofía in sutilezas,Doña Carolina,vieja sorda y servicial que de jó nuestra pava parecida a una pava,un mapuche borracho y debil mental,de apariencia patibularia,dos comensalez más o menos normales y la flor de la reunión: Doña Rosita,una vieja loca. La conversación gira en torno a un he cho macabro deque Rosita ha sido testigo:porque parece que ha sido la úni ca el momento en que a su pobre vecina un hombre con un gran cuchillo la descueró integramente.-
- Y,gritaba su vecina, Doña Rosita?
- Imaginese como para no gritar,la pelaba viva! Y eso no estodo,despues la llevé hasta el mar y la tiró a la orilla para que se la llevarjel agua. Hay si oir gritar a esa mujer partía el alma señor usted viera!
-Porque no avisó a la policia,Rosita?
-Para q ue? Se acuerda cuando la pelaron a su prima?,bueno fuí a hacer la denuncia y me dijeron que estaba loca que me dejara de cosas raras porque e sino me iban a encerrar,fijese. No,yo no aviso más a la gente esa.Despues de un rato la conversación gira sobre el enviado de dios,un prójimo que usa lo poderes que le hadado el Señor para curar la sordera,la mudez,la parálisis, etc.,luego pasa el platillo. Parece que el negocio no es más malo que otros del monton. La publicidad de los pasquines es extraordinaria y la credulidad de la gente tambien,pero eso si,de las cosas que veía Doña Rosita se reían con toda la tranquilidad del mundo.

Facsimiles of "La Gioconda's Smile," from Che's manuscript
of *The Motorcycle Diaries*.

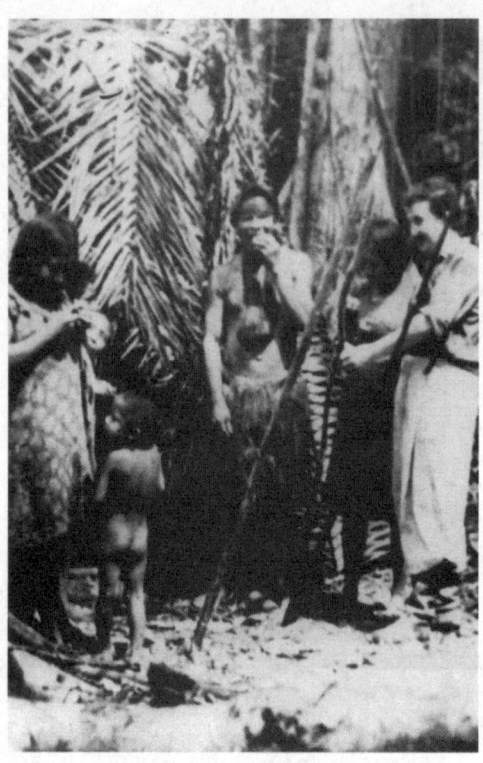

Alberto Granado with members of the Yagua indigenous community.

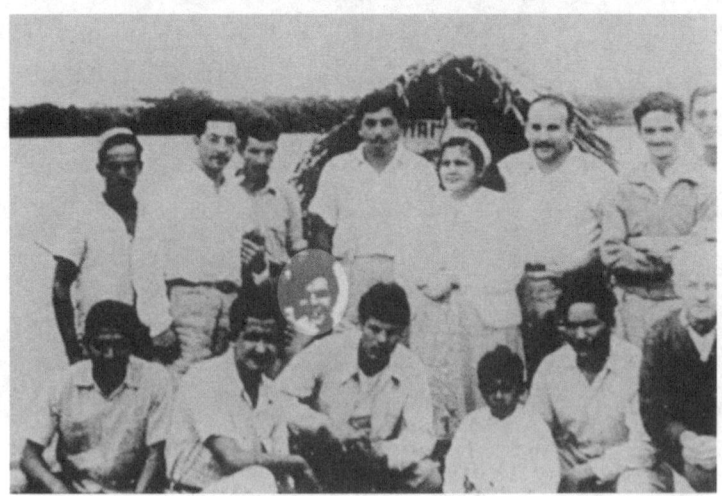

In front of the *Mambo Tango* raft.

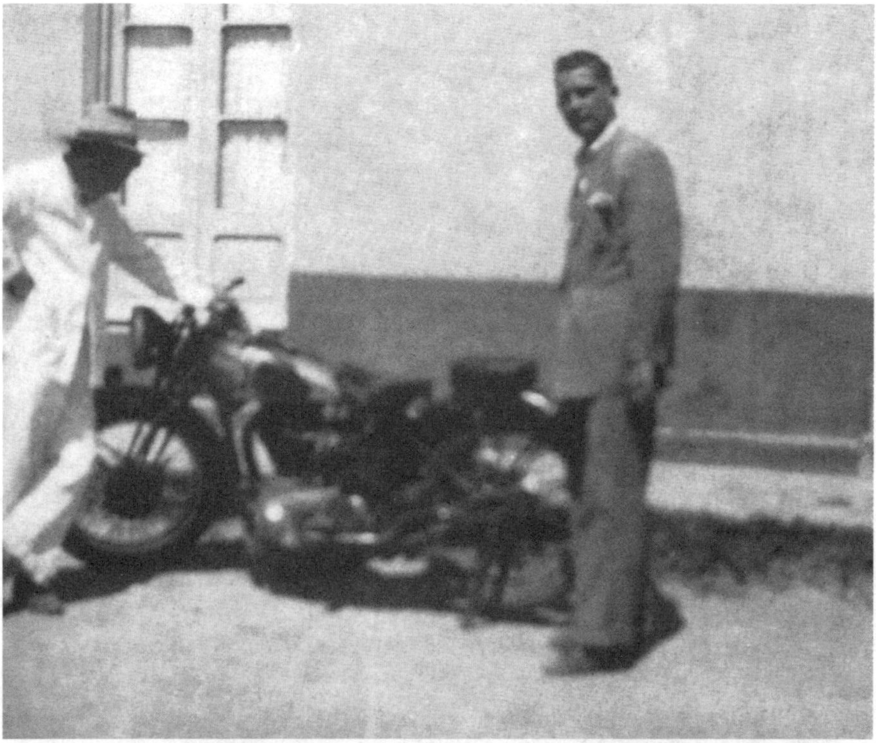

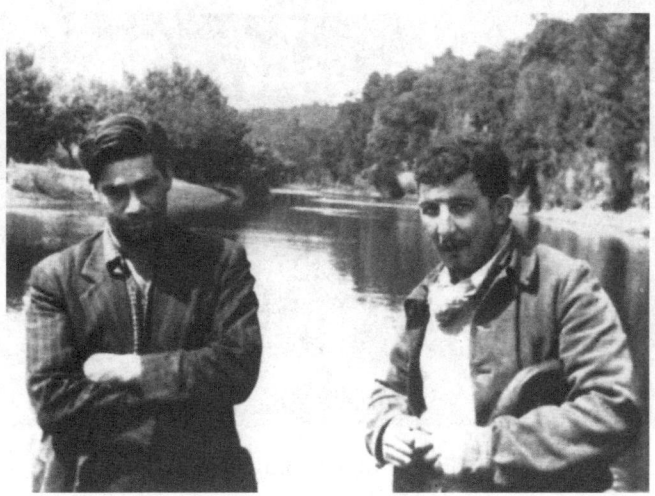

The famous "La Poderosa II" motorcycle.

Alberto Granado (right) with a Peruvian peasant

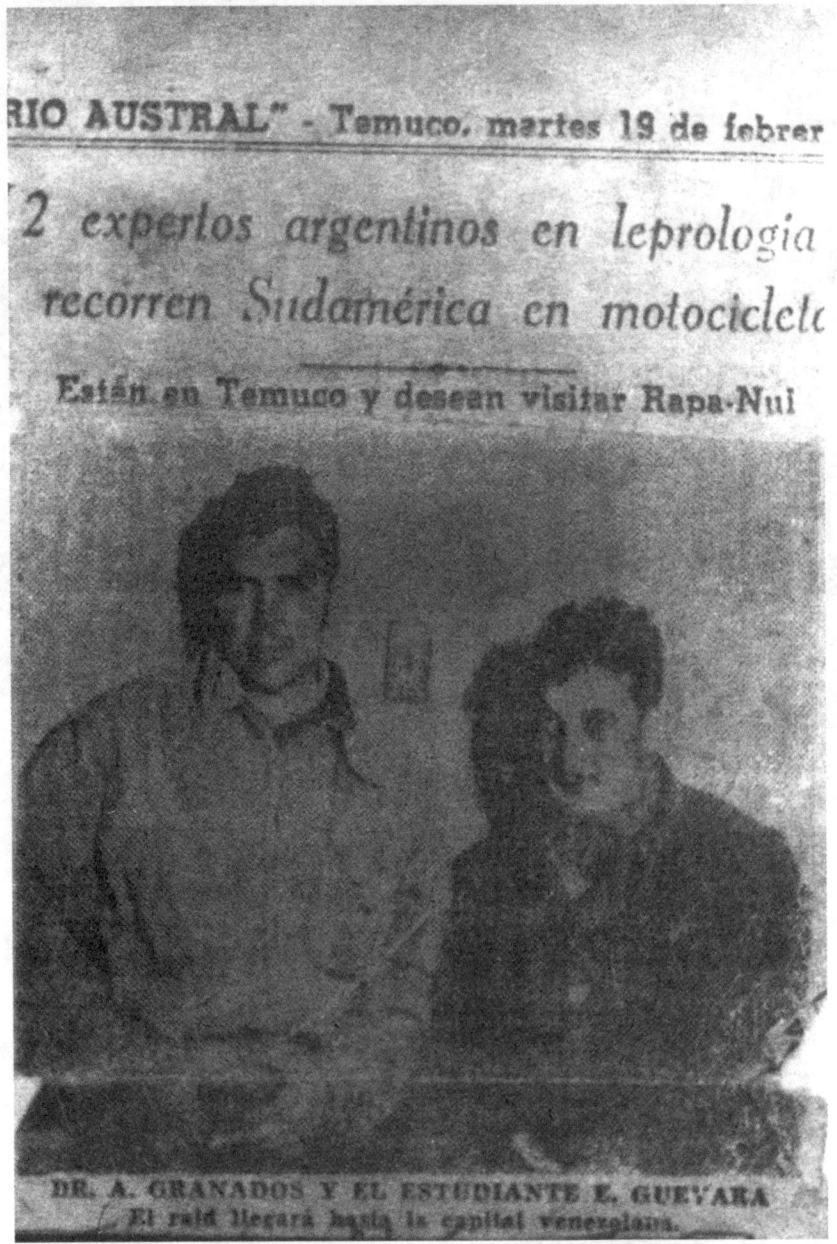

Newspaper clipping from *Austral*, February 19, 1952.

SECOND TRIP AROUND LATIN AMERICA

Excerpts from Che's *Latin America Diaries:* Otra Vez or *A Second Look at Latin America*.

Lima

I went to visit Dr. Pesce and the people from the leprosy colony.[1] Everyone greeted me most cordially.

[...]

Dr. Pesce honored us with one of his rambling, genial chats in which he touches with such assurance on so many diverse topics.

Ecuador

Guayaquil, like all these ports, is an excuse for a city that barely has its own life. It revolves around the daily succession of ships arriving and departing.

[...]

Later, I met a young guy, Maldonado, who introduced me to some medical people, including Dr. Safadi, a psychiatrist and a "bolshie" [Bolshevik] like his friend Maldonado.[2] They put me in touch with another leprosy specialist.

They have a closed colony with 13 people in fairly bad condition, for whom there is little specific treatment.

At least the hospitals are clean and not all that bad.

Panama

Nothing new, except that tomorrow I am to give a lecture on allergies, saying something about the organization of the medical faculty in Buenos

---

[1] The De Guia Leprosy Colony. Both Dr. Pesce and his assistant Zoraida Boluarte had offered support during Ernesto's first trip around Latin America with Alberto Granado, so he visited them when he returned to Lima.

[2] Dr. Jorge Maldonado Reinilla and Dr. Fortunato Safadi.

Aires. The students gave me a warm welcome at the college. I met Don Santiago Pi Suñer, the physiologist, and in another context we met Dr. Carlos Guevara Moreno, who struck me as an intelligent demagogue, knowledgeable in mass psychology but not in the dialectics of history. He is very nice and friendly and treated us with deference. He gives the impression that he knows what he's doing and where he's going, but that he wouldn't take a revolution beyond what is strictly indispensable to keep the masses content. He admires Perón. We might be able to publish two articles, one in *Siete*, the other in the Sunday supplement of *Panamá-América*.

[...]

I gave the famous lecture to an audience of 12, including Dr. Santiago Pi Suñer, for $25. I wrote an article about the Amazon, $20, and one about Machu-Picchu, probably $25.

We're going to move to a place that's rent free. We met a young painter, not a bad guy.

Costa Rica, at the "Golfito" port

The famous *Pachuca*, which transports *pachucos* (bums), is leaving port tomorrow, Sunday. We now have beds. The hospital is comfortable and you can get proper medical attention, but its comforts vary depending on your position in the [United Fruit] Company. As always, the class spirit of the gringos is clearly evident.

San José

I didn't see the leprosarium, but I did meet two excellent people: Dr. Arturo Romero, a tremendously cultured man who due to various intrigues has been removed from the leprosarium board; and Dr. Alfonso Trejos, a researcher and a very fine person.

I visited the hospital, and just this morning, the leprosarium.

[...]

A day that left no trace: boredom, reading, weak jokes. Roy, a little old pensioner from Panama, came in for me to look at him because he thought he was going to die from a tapeworm. He has chronic salteritis.

Guatemala

Nothing new in terms of finding work. The administrative efforts at the Ministry of Public Health have failed. For now the only game in town appears to be a radio contract; although nothing's come of it yet, it looks promising. We've met no one interesting these last few days. I put on the ACTH from 8 a.m. until 2 p.m. or so in the afternoon. I'm fine.

No prospects in the near future. The *éminence grise* did not keep the appointment we made with him.

[...]

A Sunday without novelty, until the evening when I was asked to attend to one of the Cubans[3] who was complaining of severe abdominal pain. I called an ambulance and we waited in the hospital until 2 a.m., when the doctor decided it was necessary to wait before operating. We left him under observation.

Earlier, at a party in Myrna Torres's home,[4] I met a girl who was showing some interest in me and talked about the possibility of some work for 40 quetzals. We'll see.

[...]

I've had asthma these days, the last few confined to my room hardly going out at all, although yesterday (Sunday) we went with the Venezuelans and Nicanor Mujica to Amatitlán. There we got into a heavy argument, all of them against me, except for Fatty Rojo who said I don't have the moral ability to engage in a debate. Today I went to see about the possibility of work as a doctor: 80 a month, for one hour's work a day. In the IGSS they told me with utmost certainty that there are no positions.

[...]

Several days have passed, two of them at La Viña colony. A spectacular place, in a landscape similar to the Sierras Grandes in Córdoba, and human material to be worked into shape. But they lack that essential ingredient: the desire to pay for a doctor of their own.

[...]

---

[3] This is the first mention in the diary of the Cubans who mounted the attack on the Moncada and Bayamo barracks in July 1953, some of whom were then in Guatemala. Ernesto had contact with them through Myrna Torres, the daughter of Edelberto Torres, who was a friend of Hilda Gadea. Ernesto later married Hilda in Mexico.

[4] Myrna Torres recalls this party was on Sunday January 24, 1954, and the girl was a teacher, Norma Cabrera.

After confusion over the matter of introductions, I went to the farm with Peñalver, who rather demagogically proposed me for the job. The director asked me how much I wanted, and I kept it low at 100 quetzals for twice a week, on the condition they spend 25 a month on laboratory equipment. I have to go back on Saturday to see what the outcome is.

The whole farm business is very murky. Answer postponed. I went to Tiquisate and it didn't go well, but there's some hope of not such a good job, with board and lodging.

[…]

Today I'm in a great mood. It was Julia Mejías who introduced me to García Granados, who said he would give me a job to go to Petén for $125. I still need authorization from the union, which I'll try to get tomorrow. If it happens it'll be great […]. Tomorrow could be a day of further disappointment, or my big day in Guatemala. I am optimistic.

Now I'm not so optimistic — far from it. I spoke with Sibaja, but he paid me no attention. At 4 p.m. tomorrow he'll tell me once and for all whether he's been able to influence the head of the union. On another front, tomorrow Lily will speak to her brother. It will probably come to nothing again. We'll see. The Geografía work continues, although today I just wandered around, not doing a lot.

[…]

Two more days to add to this concert of complaints, but with a couple of positive results. Yesterday was the visit to the former house of Lily's famous brother, ostentatious but with a good consulting room and some sort of a laboratory. The woman is Italian, and has sparked my desire to travel to Europe. They have something Indo-Americans are missing. I had a touch of asthma that started to get worse, but I swallowed a few of Ross's pills and it stopped.

[…]

Two more days in the sun; everything and nothing has happened. The job is still unresolved, although my impression is that it's mine. I spoke to the union boss, who said he would submit a list of questions to the contractor.

Two more days with nothing fully resolved. I'm now saying I'm going to El Petén, although I don't have the slightest assurance that this is the case.

I'm at the point of making a list of what I will need […]. I am desperate to go. Perhaps by Monday everything will be settled.

[…]

Bad news yet again. This is the story that never ends. The son of a bitch Andrade wouldn't even see me; this morning he made me ask myself a couple of times what I really wanted to do. I'm really up in the air and don't know what to do.

[…]

Enthusiasm depends on health and circumstances; both have been failing me. The Petén job seems more and more remote. The letter has already gone to Dr. Aguilar but, of course, I haven't received an answer. The whole thing is fucked. I don't know what the hell to do […]. I feel like pissing off — perhaps to Venezuela.

More days, if not ripe with results, then at least with promises. From Tiquisate, no news. From Buenos Aires, news of the death of my aunt Sara. From El Petén, I've stopped counting on it. From the boarding house, that I have to pay up. From the gringo, that he doesn't like the food at his new boarding house, and that if it doesn't improve we can swap places […]. From Sra. de Holst, that I should go and live with her. That's a précis of my recent life. I'm practicing at the Sanidad laboratory in case they call me to Tiquisate — otherwise I'm just waiting to see what happens. I've promised to pay the boarding house by Saturday for at least a month, which is just two days away, but I don't know where that cash will come from.

[…]

Days continue to pass, but I no longer care. Maybe I'll change my mind about the thing with Helenita Leyva, maybe not. Either way, I know things will sort themselves out, and I'm no longer doing my head in.

In terms of work, nothing can be done about the residency permit until after Easter; the minister for health said I could ask around, and I know there's work at Livingston on the Atlantic coast, which Helenita will ask about for me on Monday. Hilda says she will ask about a job at the OAS [Organization of American States]. We'll see what comes of all this, but I don't have many illusions. My mind is made up, and one of these days I'll write to China and see what they have to say.

[…]

The invaders believed they only had to say the word and the people would rise up as one to follow them, and that's why they parachute-dropped weapons, but the people immediately rallied to defend Árbenz. Although the invading troops were blocked and defeated on all fronts until they were pushed back beyond Chiquimula near the Honduran border, the pirate airplanes kept attacking the battlefronts and towns, always coming from bases in Honduras and Nicaragua. Chiquimula was heavily bombed and bombs also fell on Guatemala City, injuring several people and killing a three-year-old little girl.

My own life unfolded as follows: First I reported to the youth brigades of the Alliance where we stayed for several days until the minister of public health [Dr. Carlos Tejedas] sent me to the Maestro Health Center where I am billeted. I volunteered for the front but they wouldn't even look at me.

[...]

Today, Saturday, June 26, the minister came by when I had gone to see Hilda [Gadea]; she gave me hell because I wanted to ask him to send me to the front [...].

[...]

My personal situation is more or less that I'll be expelled from the little hospital where I am now, probably tomorrow, because I have been renamed "Chebol"[5] and the repression is coming.[6]

Mexico

Several days have passed, and in general I can say that apart from the bitterness at not being able to study anything but medicine during the day, I've managed to achieve some things. On Monday I'll see about a medical position, on Wednesday one of the others; in the meantime I'll continue with photography and getting to know people.

[...]

I am still working discreetly at photography, but you need to be fit and always on the go. I'm establishing myself at the hospitals and I think I might

---

5   Che (a common Argentine form of address) combined with Bol(shevik).

6   In June 1954 the CIA backed a military coup against democratically elected President Jacobo Arbenz. Ernesto, and many supporters of the Arbenz government's social reforms, had to leave Guatemala. He arrived in Mexico in September.

have work, although not in the Institute of Nutrition. I've moved to a decent room in the center of the city, costing me 100 pesos a month.

[…]

The photography isn't going badly, and medicine looks promising. I'm earning a living […]. Right now my intellectual life is nonexistent, except for some reading at night and a tiny bit of daily study.

[…]

A bit of water has passed under the bridge. In general, things are as follows: To survive, I really have nothing but photography, and it doesn't pay enough. This week I took roughly 60 photos, meaning a similar number of pesos (not inconsiderable), but half of them failed because of a blurred roll of film. In the medical arena, I'm working three days at each of the hospitals: the Children's and the General. At the General hospital I'm working on Pisani's food digestion, and the Children's hospital asked me to present a work plan, of which I already have an outline.

[…]

I'm busy at the hospital in the mornings, although I don't do anything, and there's not enough time in the evening to deliver the photos, so I'm in debt.

[…]

Some fairly important things have happened over the last few days. Out in the street one day I met the head of the Agencia Latina, a doctor,[7] who took a liking to me and gave me a provisional job as a correspondent. I dug out the things from *Panamá-América* and got a bit of money for them, not much, but probably enough to get by. The photography is a slow road. I am falling into debt, but I'm also owed money. I'm working at the hospital with no idea where it will get me.

[…]

The days follow one another in rapid succession. I'm doing a lot of work on allergies and I'm in close contact with the doctors.

In general I think I'll keep at it, in the full knowledge that triumphs come hand in hand with hard knocks. On Monday I have an interview at the Agencia

---

[7]   The doctor was Alfonso Pérez Vizcaino. This was to cover the Pan-American Games, which took place in Mexico between March 12 and 16, 1955. Ernesto was an accredited Agencia Latina reporter from January 31 to December 31, 1955.

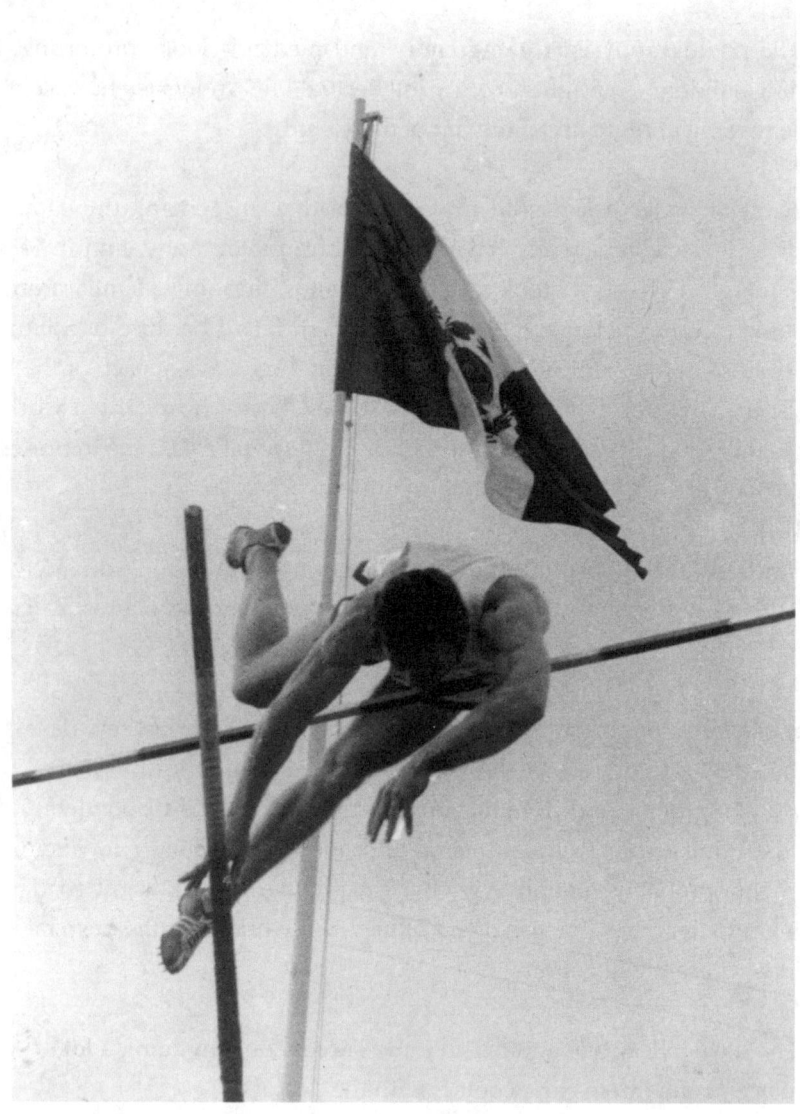

Photograph taken by Ernesto when he was working as a photo journalist during the 1955 Pan-American Games.

Latina to see if I can get work there. I'm doing less and less photography because traveling all over the city for nothing is exhausting.

[...]

Work at the hospital goes well, although every day I realize that outside of allergies, I don't know the first thing about medicine. I'm treating two patients at each hospital. My hands are tied at the Children's hospital and I can't really do anything, but at the General I have a lot of freedom. I'd quite like to do some electrophoresis[8] experiments but don't know what results I'll get.

[...]

The year is coming to an end and a change in my economic prospects seems certain. Science-wise I continue as before, working on food digestion and preparing to work on blood electrophoresis with Urbach equipment. At the Children's hospital, they want me to do some experimental work, with a wage and everything. I'm still working at the Agencia Latina, but I haven't been paid anything yet. My studies are at a standstill: I read very little medicine, a little more literature, but hardly ever write.

[...]

In the scientific field, I have great hopes, but nothing has yet materialized. I started studying how to do electrophoresis with filter paper, and I hope to start working on it in a week or two.

[...]

My homemade electrophoresis machine works slowly, while the other work is virtually at a standstill. Dr. Cortés and I are looking after a patient who I believe should improve rapidly; I charge her 20 pesos a consult. I hope the coming week will be eventful [...].

My patient's condition worsened. I did some further tests and she is sensitive to various foods, so I have taken her off them. Despite everything I still have no money, and there's no way of making ends meet [...].

Now that the Pan-American Games[9] are approaching, I'll have to work like a slave and put hospital work to the side. My patient is stable, exactly where I left her. I think I have broken with Hilda for good after a melodramatic scene. I fancy a girl who's a chemist: she's not particularly intelligent

---

8   The motion of proteins (electrically charged molecules) in the presence of an electrical field.

9   The Pan-American Games were held March 12-16, 1955, in Mexico.

and fairly ignorant, but she has an appealing freshness and fantastic eyes. I'll present a paper at the Allergy Congress in April on cutaneous tests with food digestion.

[...]

Scientifically, I've promised to finish a paper for the Allergy Congress, which I think I can do. They have invited me to Nuevo Laredo, near the border with the gringos, but it would be for two years' work and I'm not up for it. My plans are simpler: Until March I'll do the allergy work and present the paper; in May, June and July I'll travel around Mexico from north to south and east to west; in July-August I'll go to Veracruz and wait for a ship to Cuba or Europe; if that's not possible, I'll be in Caracas by December. We'll see how it all works out.

A lot of water has passed under my bridge. [...] I'm now an intern at the hospital. It happened like this: I went to León, Guanajuato, and presented my paper, "Cutaneous Investigations with Semi-Digested Food Antigens."[10] The paper was a minor success, and Salazar Mallén, head of Mexican allergy research, commented on it. It will now be published in the journal *Alergia*. Salazar Mallén promised me some financial help for research work and a position as an intern at the General Hospital, but that remains to be seen.

[...]

After many adventures I am now established at the General Hospital and working fairly hard, although without much structure. The food is not great: if I eat it I get asthma, if I don't I go hungry. Salazar Mallén pays me 150 pesos [...].

[...]

A scientific event was the appearance of my first medical paper as sole author, in the journal *Alergia*: "Cutaneous Investigations with Semi-Digested Food Antigens"; passable.

In physiology, I have become a cat surgeon.

[...]

---

10   A paper presented at the Ninth National Congress of Allergists, held at the León School of Medicine, University of Guanajuato, April 25-30, 1955. The paper was later published in the Revista Iberoamericana de Alergología, Mexico City, May 1955.

I'm a little more focused on my studies: reading only on allergies and studying a bit of English and algebra. I'm researching only three matters, with another one maybe in the future: histamines in the blood, histamines in tubercular lung tissue and progesterone in relation to histamines. I am thinking of doing some serum electrophoresis. On another topic, I've bought a camera to replace the one that was stolen, and I'm learning to touch-type. I still don't know whether I'll get work at the United Nations; the idea repels me but the money is attractive.

[...]

A long time has passed and there have been many events not yet recounted. I'll just note the most important one. Since February 15, 1956, I'm a father: Hilda Beatriz Guevara is my firstborn.

I belong to the Roca del CE group of Mexico.

Five jobs I was offered all fell through, so I signed up as a cameraman in a small company and my progress in cinematography has been rapid. My plans for the future are unclear but I hope to finish a couple of research projects. This could be an important year for my future. I've already given up hospitals. I'll write soon with more details.[11]

---

[11]   These were the last notes in this diary. On November 25, 1956, Che set sail from Tuxpan, Mexico, on the *Granma* cabin cruiser headed to Cuba to initiate the struggle against the Batista dictatorship.

El Congreso de Alergistas

Trascendentales Ponencias se han Sometido a Estudio

Múltiples y abundantes comentarios han provocado las ponencias presentadas en el IX Congreso Nacional de Alergistas, pues los trabajos que médicos especialistas de todo el país han leído ante sus colegas encierran adelantos y experiencias personales que se ponen al alcance de todos los alergistas que buscan la abundancia de conocimientos como piedra de toque para la mejor atención y cura de los enfermos.

En efecto, las dos sesiones de trabajo celebradas a la fecha abundan en ponencias trascendentales que provocaron los lógicos comentarios de aprobación, declaraciones, etc., entre los numerosos médicos congregistas. Fue especialmente notable el trabajo del doctor Oswaldo Arias, Director de la Escuela Médico Militar, quien leyó un trabajo que pone al corriente a los alergistas del país, sobre el uso del ungüento de Hidrocortisona en la dermatología, médicamente que, como informamos ayer, se ha empleado por primera vez en nuestro país. El Presidente del Congreso, doctor López Sanabria, presentó, por su parte, otra interesantísima ponencia sobre la Alergia por alimentos.

El Congreso, evento científico de gran resonancia, será clausurado hoy a las 13.00 horas, en la ceremonia de clausura, se entregarán diplomas a todos los congresistas, y a los médicos alumnos del Sexto Curso Anual sobre Alergia que tuvo por sede a nuestra ciudad.

La última sesión habrá de verificarse en el Aula B de la Facultad de Medicina, conforme al programa que sigue:

9 horas.— "Hongos atmosféricos en la región medio occidental de la República Mexicana". Por el doctor Arturo Blackaller.

9.30 horas.— "Investigaciones cutáneas con antígenos alimenticios digeridos", por el doctor Ernesto Guevara, de la República Argentina.

10.00 horas.— "Dermatitis Atópica y su relación con antigenos inhalables". Dr. David Gordillo Hernández.

10.30 horas.— "Dermatitis Atópica". Revisión de cien casos, por el doctor Fernando Martínez C.

11.00 horas.— "Actinodermia", "Dermatitis Solar". Su tratamiento, por el doctor Raymundo Arroyave.

11.30 horas.— "Pólenes atmosféricos en la región medio occidental de la República Mexicana". Por el doctor Arturo Blackaller.

12.00 horas.— "Estudio de trescientos niños alérgicos". Dr. Luis Gómez Orozco.

13.00 horas.— Clausura del curso y del Congreso y entrega de diplomas.

Decisions of the Ninth National Congress of Allergists, April 1955, Mexico.

SABADO 30

9.00 Hs.—SESION DE TRABAJOS DEL CONGRESO. (Aula B).

9.00 Hs.—HONGOS ATMOSFERICOS EN LA REGION MEDIO OCCIDENTAL DE LA REP. MEXICANA.—Dr. Arturo Blackaller.

9.30 Hs.—INVESTIGACIONES CUTANEAS CON ANTIGENOS ALIMENTICIOS DIGERIDOS.—Dr. Ernesto Guevara.

10.00 Hs.—DERMATITIS ATOPICA Y SU RELACION CON ANTIGENOS INHALABLES.—Dr. David Gordillo Hernández.

10.30 Hs.—DERMATITIS ATOPICA.—Revisión de 100 casos. —Dr Fernando Martínez C.

11.00 Hs.—ACTINODERMIA. --DERMATITIS SOLAR.— SU TRATAMIENTO.—Dr. Raymundo Arroyave.

11.30 Hs.—POLENES ATMOSFERICOS EN LA REGION MEDIO OCCIDENTAL DE LA REP. MEXICANA.— Dr. Arturo Blackaller.

12.00 Hs.—ESTUDIO DE 300 NIÑOS ALERGICOS.—Dr. Luis Gómez Orozco.

13.00 Hs.—Clausura del curso y del congreso. ENTREGA DE DIPLOMAS.

N o t a s :

Program of activities of the Ninth National Congress of Allergists.

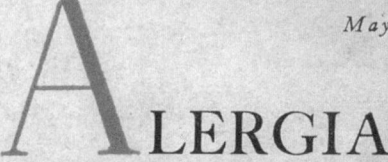

Vol. II, Num. 4   *Mayo, 1955**

ALERGIA

REVISTA IBEROAMERICANA DE ALERGOLOGIA

Director General: DR. MARIO SALAZAR MALLEN - México, D. F., México

D i r e c t o r e s
a s o c i a d o s   DR. GUIDO RUIZ MORENO
Buenos Aires, Argentina
DR. CARLOS CANSECO JR.
Monterrey, Nuevo León

R e d a c t o r e s   ARGENTINA: Dr. A. E. Bachmann,
Dr. J. E. F. Dumm, Dr. J. Martorelli, Dr. M. A. Solari.
BRASIL: Dr. E. Mendes. CUBA: Dr. J. Quintero Fossas.
CHILE: Dr. E. Díaz Carrasco. ECUADOR: Dr. P. Naranjo
Vargas. ESPAÑA: Dr. B. Sánchez Cuenca. MÉXICO: Dr. J.
Cueva, Dr. F. Martínez Cortés.

SUMARIO

Alergia magazine, featuring an article by Ernesto Guevara and
edited by Dr. Mario Salazar Mallén, May 1955.

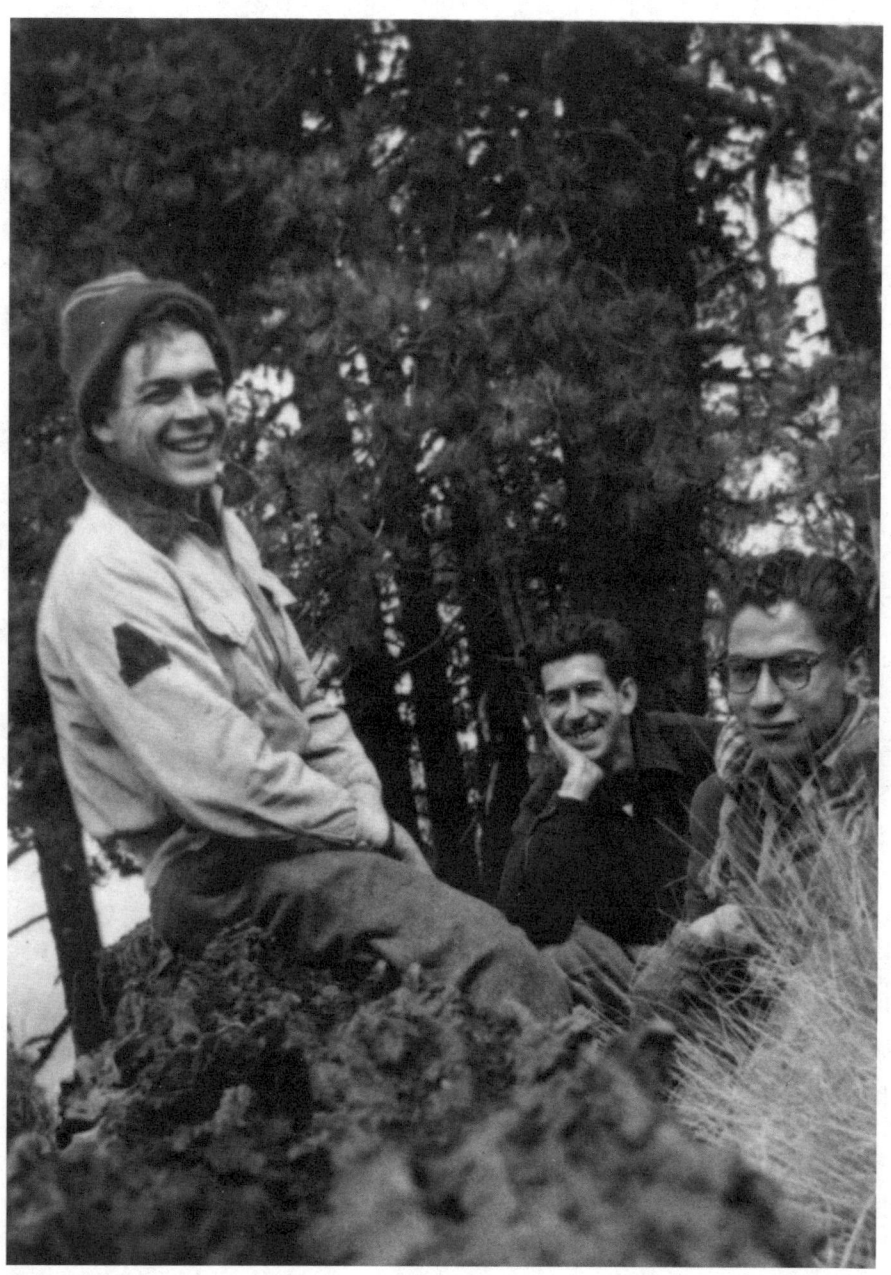

Ernesto and friends in Mexico.

LETTERS FROM TRAVELS IN LATIN AMERICA (1954-1956)

Letter from Ernesto to his mother from Mexico [Approximately early November 1954]

Vieja, my *vieja*, [*Old Lady*]

(I confused you with the date)

[...]

Even [Aunt] Beatriz is engaging in reprisals, and those telegrams she used to send no longer come.

To tell you about my life is to repeat myself because I'm not doing anything new. Photography is bringing in enough to live on and there is really no basis for believing I might be able to give it up anytime soon, although I'm working every morning as a researcher in two hospitals. I think the best thing for me would be to slip into an unofficial job as a country doctor, somewhere near the capital. This would make it easier to devote my time to medicine for a few months. I'm doing this because I'm perfectly aware of how much I learned about allergies with Pisani. Now I have compared notes with people who've studied in the United States, and who are no fools with regard to orthodox knowledge, I think that Pisani's method is light years ahead. I want to get practical experience with the nuts and bolts of his systems so that I can land on my feet wherever that might be [...].

I'm slaving away here, busy every morning in the hospital and in the afternoons and Sundays I work as a photographer, while at night I study a bit. I think I mentioned I'm in a good apartment, I cook my own food and do everything myself, as well as bathing every day thanks to the unlimited supply of hot water.

As you can see, I'm changing in this aspect, but otherwise I'm the same because I don't wash my clothes very often, and wash them badly when I do, and I still don't earn enough to pay a laundry.

The scholarship is a dream I've given up on, as I had thought that in such a large country all you had to do was ask for something and it was done. You know that I have always been inclined to make drastic decisions, and here the pay is great. Everyone is lazy, but they don't get in the way when other people get things done, so I've got a free rein either here or in the country where I might go next. Naturally, this doesn't make me lose sight of my goal, which is Europe, where I'm planning to go no matter what happens.

As for the United States, I haven't lost an ounce of hostility, but I do want to check out New York, at least. I'm not in the least worried about what might happen and know that I'll leave just as anti-Yankee as when I arrive (that's if I do get in).

I'm happy that people are waking up a bit, although I don't know what direction they are moving in. Anyway, the truth is that Argentina is as insular as you can get even though in general terms the picture we get from here seems to suggest that they are taking important steps forward and that the country will be perfectly able to defend itself from the crisis the Yankees are about to set off by dumping their surplus food […].

Communists don't have your sense of friendship but, among themselves, it is the same or better than yours. I have seen this very clearly and, in the chaos of Guatemala after the government was overthrown and it was every man for himself, the communists maintained their faith and comradeship and they constitute the only group that continued to work there.

I think they deserve respect and sooner or later I'll join the party. What mainly holds me back from doing so, for the moment, is that I'm desperate to travel around Europe and I couldn't do this if I had to submit to a rigid discipline.

Vieja, till Paris

Letter from Ernesto to his mother from Mexico [no date, probably around the end of 1954]

Vieja, my *vieja*,

It's true, I've been too lazy, but the real guilty party, as always, is Don Dinero [Mr. Money]. Anyway, the end of this wretched financial year of 1954—part of which has treated me beautifully (like your face) — coin-

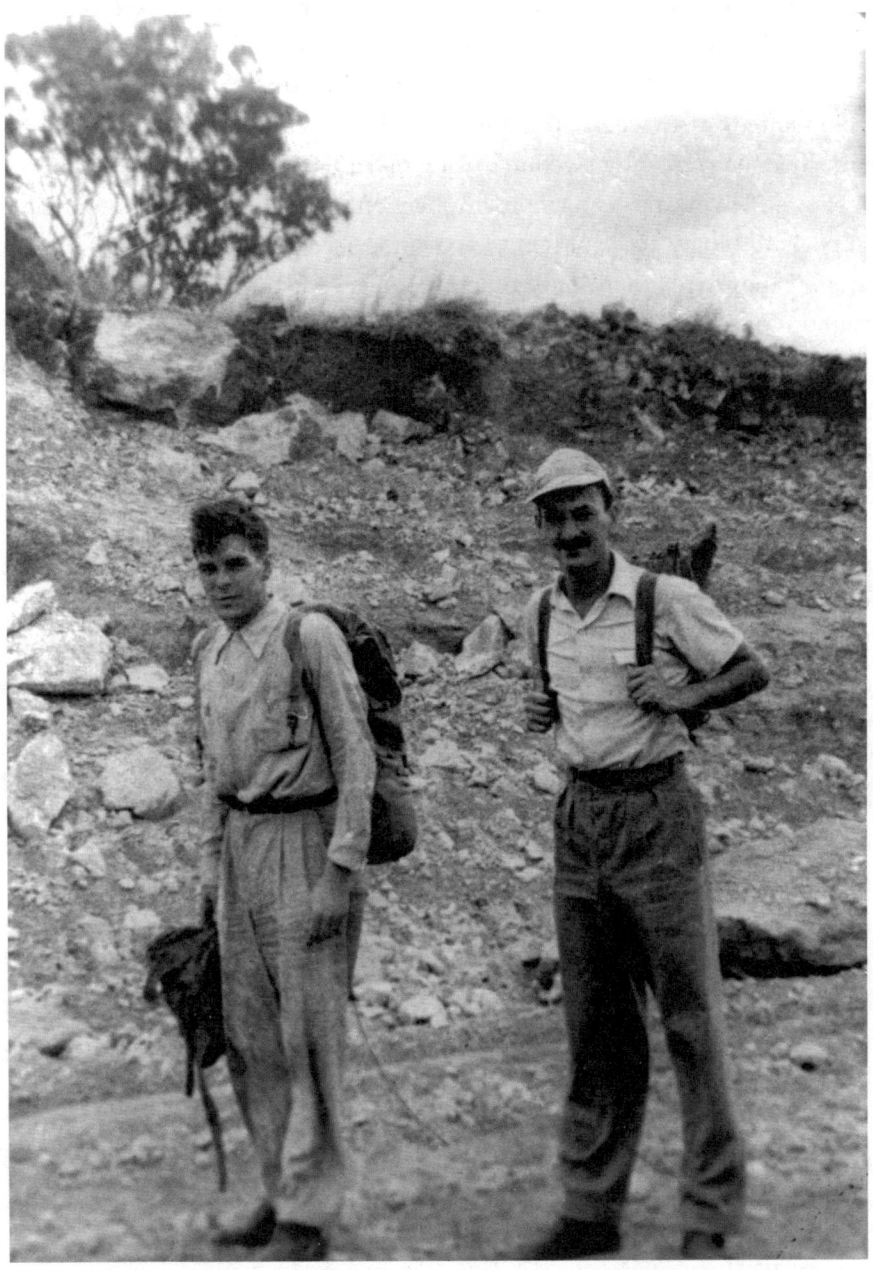

Ernesto with his travel companion Gualo García during his second trip
around Latin America. Costa Rica, 1953.

cides with the end of my chronic hunger. I'm working as an editor at the Agencia Latina for 700 Mexican pesos a month (equivalent to 700 Argentine pesos), enough to live on with the added bonus that I work for only three hours, three days a week. I can therefore spend whole mornings at the hospital, where I am creating swellings using Pisani's method. [...]

I'm still working as a photographer, but also spending time on more important things, like "studying," and some strange little things that pop up around the place. There's not much left over, but this December I hope to round it out to 1,000 and with a bit of luck, we'll do a bit of photography at the end of the coming year (at the beginning, I meant to write). Contrary to what you might think, I'm no worse than the majority of photographers here, and the best among my compañeros, although yes, in this group you only need one eye to win the crown.

My immediate plans involve staying some six months or so in Mexico, which I find interesting and like a lot, and in this time apply, by the way, for a visa to visit "the children of the super power," as Arévalo calls them. If I get it, I'll go. If not, I'll see what other concrete plans I can make. I haven't abandoned the idea of slipping behind the Iron Curtain to see what's happening there. As you see, there's nothing new since earlier reports.

I'm very enthusiastic about the scientific research, which I'm capitalizing on because it won't last. I have two research projects on the run and may start on a third — all related to allergies — and very slowly I'm collecting material for a little book that will come to light (if ever) in a couple of years with the pretentious title, The Role of the Doctor in Latin America. I can speak with some authority on the subject, considering that, although I don't know much about medicine, I do have Latin America sized up. Of course, apart from a general plan and three or four chapters, I've written nothing, but time is on my side.

With regard to the changes in my thinking, which is becoming sharper, I promise you that it will only be for a short time. What you are so afraid of can be reached in two ways: the positive one, when you convince someone directly, or the negative one, through a disillusionment with everything. I came along the second path, only to be immediately convinced that it is essential to follow the first. The way that the gringos treat Latin America (remember that the gringos are Yankees) was making me feel increasingly indignant, but at the same time I studied the reasons for their actions and found a scientific explanation.

Then came Guatemala and everything that is difficult to recount. I saw how the object of one's enthusiasm was diluted by what those gentlemen decided, how a new tale of red guilt and criminality was concocted, and how the same treacherous Guatemalans set about propagating the story to get a few crumbs from the table of the new order. I can't tell you the precise moment I put reasoning aside and acquired something like faith, not even approximately, as the journey was long and there were many backward steps. [...]

Letter from Ernesto to his mother from Mexico [Approximately October 1956]

Dear Mamá,

Your lousy son, who, besides being the son of a bad mother, is not a good-for-nothing; he's like Paul Muni[12] who says what he says in that tragic voice, and then disappears into the lengthening shadows to the sound of evocative music. My current profession is that of a grasshopper, here today, gone tomorrow, etc.,

My relatives... well, I haven't been to see them because of this (and also, I confess, because I probably have more in common with a whale than with a bourgeois married couple employed in the kinds of worthy institutions I would wipe from the face of the earth if I got the chance to do so. I don't want you to think that this is just a passing aversion; it's real mistrust. Lezica has shown that we speak different languages and have no common points of reference.) I have given you this lengthy bracketed explanation because, after my opening line, I thought you might imagine I'm on the way to a becoming a *morfa-burgués*.[13] Being too lazy to start over and remove the paragraph, I embarked on a lengthy explanation that now strikes me as rather unconvincing. Full stop, new paragraph.

---

[12]   The reference is to the film *I Am a Fugitive from a Chain Gang*, in which Paul Muni played the leading role.

[13]   Argentine slang meaning a lazy bourgeois who does nothing but eat

Within a month, Hilda will go to visit her family in Peru, taking advantage of the fact that she is no longer a political criminal but [now regarded as] a somewhat misguided representative of the admirable and anticommunist party the APRA [Alianza Popular Revolucionaria Americana]. For my part, I'm in the process of changing the focus of my studies: whereas previously I devoted myself for better or worse to medicine, and spent my spare time informally studying Saint Carlos [Marx], this new stage of my life demands that I change the priorities. Now Saint Carlos is primordial; he is the axis and will remain so for however many years the spheroid has room for me on its outer mantle. Medicine is more or less a trivial and passing pursuit, except for one small area on which I'm thinking of writing more than one substantive study — the kind that causes bookstore basements to tremble beneath its weight.

As you'll recall, and if you don't remember I'll remind you now, I was working on a book on the role of the doctor, etc., of which I only finished a couple of chapters that whiffed of some newspaper serial with a title like *Bodies and Souls*.[14] They were nothing more than poorly written rubbish, displaying a thorough ignorance of the fundamental issues, so I decided to study. Again, to write it, I had to reach a series of conclusions that were kicking against my essentially adventurous trajectory, so I decided to deal with the main things first, to pit myself against the order of things, shield on my arm, the whole fantasy, and then, if the windmills don't crack open my nut, I'll get down to writing.

I owe [sister] Celia the letter of praise I will write after this if I have time. The others are in debt to me as the last word has been mine, even with [Aunt] Beatriz. Tell her that the papers arrive like clockwork and that they give me a very good idea of all the government's beautiful deeds. I cut out the articles carefully, following the example of my *pater*, and now Hilda is emulating her *mater*. A kiss for everyone, with all the appropriate additions and a reply — negative or positive, but convincing — about the Guatemalan.[15]

Now all that remains is the final part of the speech, which refers to the man, which could be titled: "What next?" Now comes the tough part, *vieja*,

---

14   *Corps et âmes [Bodies and Souls]* was a book written by the French writer Maxence Van der Meersch.

15   This was one of Che's friends who had arrived in Argentina as a political refugee after the coup in Guatemala.

the part I've never shunned and always enjoyed. The sky has not darkened, the stars have not fallen out of the sky, nor have there been terrible floods or hurricanes; the signs are good. They augur victory. But if they are wrong — and in the end even the gods can make mistakes — I think I'll be able to say, like a poet you don't know: "I shall carry beneath the earth only the sorrow of an unfinished song." To avoid pre-mortem pathos, this letter will appear when things get really hot, and then you'll know that your son, in some sun-drenched land in the Americas, is swearing at himself for not having studied enough surgery to help a wounded man, and cursing the Mexican government for not letting him perfect his already respectable marksmanship so he could knock over puppets with better results. The struggle will be with our backs to the wall, as in the hymns, until victory or death.

Another kiss for you, with all the love of a farewell that refuses to be a final one.

Your son

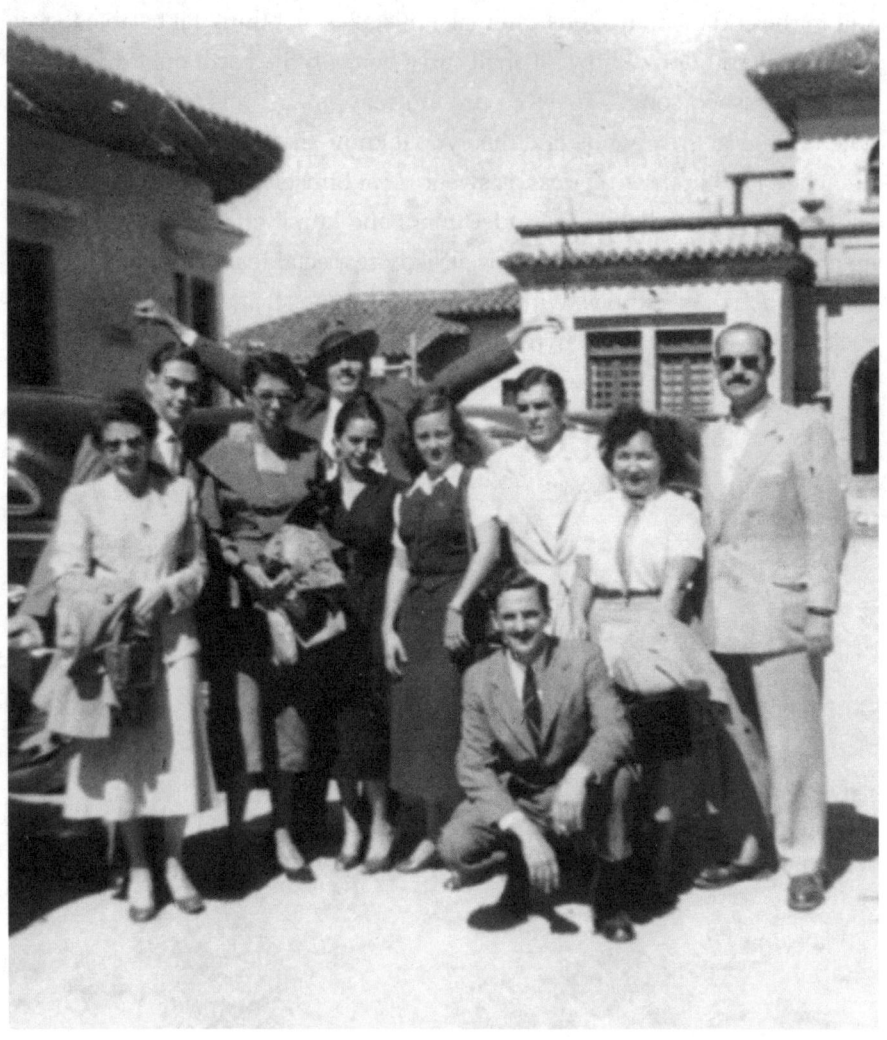

Ernesto (standing third from the right and Hilda Gadea (second from the right).

THE ROLE OF THE DOCTOR IN LATIN AMERICA*

I'm collecting material for a little book that will come to light (if ever) in a couple of years with the pretentious title, The Role of the Doctor in Latin America. *I can speak with some authority on the subject, considering that, although I don't know much about medicine, I do have Latin America sized up. Of course, apart from a general plan and three or four chapters, I've written nothing, but time is on my side.*

From a letter Ernesto sent his mother from Mexico at the end of 1954.

When initiating the struggle for the people's health, as a first step doctors should investigate what possibilities already exist in their complex surroundings. Earlier analyses have shown that facilities vary in different regions, countries, social classes and ethnic groups, and doctors must respond accordingly.

The struggle should always be expressed within a general framework that guarantees success and that leads doctors to win first the confidence and then the affection of those for whom they are medically responsible. Even though the problem can only be outlined in general terms, it should be noted that a doctor's first weapon is flexibility. Flexibility — without any very obvious probing — will allow a doctor to gain the respect of the population generally. Naturally, the conditions of struggle will vary greatly, but doctors should always take this first step along the path of consolidation.

One of the first pitfalls to be avoided is offered by colleagues and others in related professions — in small towns, a rival doctor or the pharmacist; in larger towns, a variety of colleagues and specialists. In any case, the first skirmish will always be waged on the monetary front. After a doctor has demonstrated that he is absolutely impregnable to bribes, he will be subjected to harsher attacks. Good use should be made of this period between

---

*   The following is an excerpt from Ernesto's unpublished manuscript, written between 1954 and 1956.

armed neutrality and open warfare. Later, war should be waged not only against the commercial disgraces of the profession but also against deficiencies of other kinds.

The struggle to obtain better working conditions for workers and adequate medical attention will easily lead doctors to clash with the established authorities in the sector, who are always lickspittles responding to the orders of those who hold the purse strings in the area, and with whom the authorities are sometimes confused. All activities should be carried out taking into account local public opinion supporting the popular cause that is being defended; this is where doctors should use their abilities as psychologists to the utmost — above all, in those places where the struggle must be waged directly against capital, without the help of any labor laws. Strikes are very hard to organize, unless the pretext is of such seriousness that it is understood even by those with a low level of consciousness, which is the case among the masses of workers in our continent. In general, one must be very careful not to be labeled a pro-strike doctor, because that can finish off a professional's reputation in some places.

If it is not possible to remain entirely on the sidelines, the doctor's general role will be to provide an ideological orientation, without indicating any apparent interest in the popular movement itself. Small towns contain elements that cannot be underestimated. Public opinion is much more important in such places than in the cities, and doctors should always have anecdotes to draw on to highlight the poor working and living conditions of the people they defend.

To draw up a general outline of how to conduct oneself, one must enter the battlefield armed with a good basic knowledge [of the locality]. This includes the birth rate; the infant, prenatal and general mortality rates… and, assisted by other data, the general morbidity. In cases in which there are no death or other records — which means most places in Latin America — it is a good idea to visit the local people's homes so as to gradually learn about their domestic situation.

The general picture of diseases will give you an idea of the main problems to be solved. Later, I'll go into the need for the doctor to get the inhabitants to take an active part in health care, but it can always be said that epidemic diseases — and especially endemic ones — can be combated by making correct use of the general public health system, helped by a precise understanding of the problem, explained by the doctor.

One of the doctor's most successful — although always dangerous — methods is to create health cooperatives. They are always a double-edged sword, and are usually promptly taken over by the "ladies" of the town and by other people who, in general, tend to stifle the normal development of health care. However, in those places where cooperatives must be created, this is easy to do if there is nothing else, as they will always be a step forward. Right now, to avoid being smeared as "red" — a charge which would be immediately extended to the doctor — it is not necessary to insist on having workers and peasants represented in the charitable societies, but it is important that, using a lot of common sense, the doctor start raising consciousness among the impoverished classes, making them aware of what an important role health care plays in problems of daily life.

Medically, it is essential to stress how important nutrition is in all the most common endemic diseases. Correct nutritional treatment and its corresponding success will draw attention to its importance. Doctors should remember that, in the present conditions, economic worries are primary, followed (as a complement to the former) by health care and then education.

Someone who eats well will be immediately concerned about their health care, and when that is improved — which will be a real achievement in unhealthy, marginalized communities — will then worry about the next problem: their education and that of their families.

With regard to this last aspect, while doctors should play an important counseling role, it is not a good idea for them to be in the foreground — especially in studies the nature of which will inevitably lead them to clash with the ideology of the ruling classes.

In places with deeply rooted religious traditions, one must also be careful there — at least until those who are best placed to offer systematic opposition to doctors have been neutralized.

In terms of public health, it should always be remembered that children should receive the best possible treatment. Always try to achieve success through collective action by the community rather than from the individual effort of the doctor.

The problems of individual health care are not so much the concern of the revolutionary doctor as collective health care. In terms of preventative health care, in addition to the measures that should be taken in each individual case, in accord with the established rules and regulations, doctors can set up systems for seeking and isolating diseases in the areas where they are found. When attempting to do this in an important community, Dr. Germinal Rodríguez's book *Higiene y Profilaxis* [*Health and Prophylaxis*] offers a good model.

It makes for a quite pretentious office, but the doctor needs a secretary, a lab assistant, two social workers and some volunteers in order to do this effectively. In addition to the invaluable health service it offers, a clinic of this kind also has the virtue of winning over the inhabitants to the idea of exercising their rights as citizens — which, when they get used to it, will lead many "lone wolves" to rejoin the community.

One of the points to which doctors should pay close attention is that of ensuring the government's neutrality, if nothing else. There is an apparently wide range of systems of government in Latin America, but nearly all of them share the common denominator of colonialism. This encapsulates the tragedy of the human communities now living in Latin America and has certain general features:

- control by large landowners,
- powerful authorities who oppose the people,
- control by the clergy,
- an absence of effective social laws and
- the predominance of foreign monopoly corporations.

In this panorama, with the authorities as the direct representatives of the upper social classes, doctors have to take things very slowly in order to keep the government neutral or win it over. Therefore, they should fulfill their obligations to the higher health authorities, while at the same time demanding that those authorities provide as many resources as possible. They must wage virtually a personal struggle against the exploiters, separate from the central bureaucracy, while ensuring that their medical-social activities are not seen as part of the political struggle.

It seems hardly necessary to emphasize that the doctors' work should be carried out with complete dedication, for this is what will make their ideas triumph over the inconsistent, mercenary activities of their individualistic colleagues, who view their role only as a means toward their desired goals — whether this is power (the relative power wielded by the doctor in a village), fame or money. Revolutionary doctors should always remember that it is their duty to attack whatever problems adversely affect the people, who are the only ones they should serve.

- Need for study.
- Need for exchanges with medical journals.

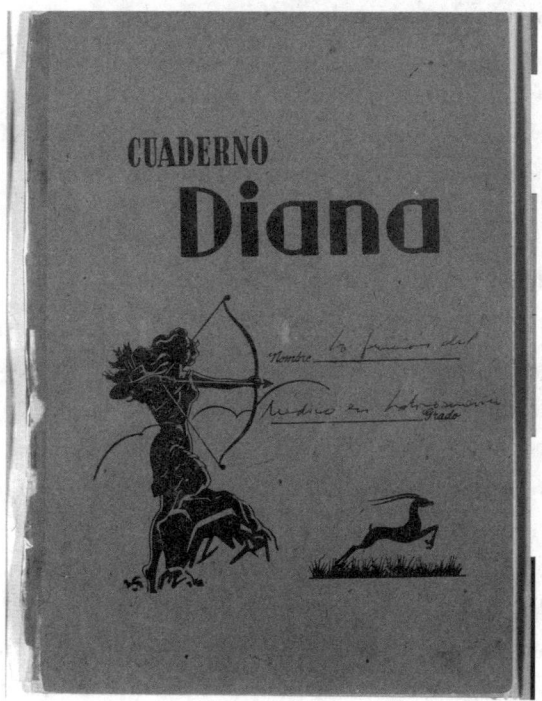

Cover of the notebook Ernesto used for drafting the book he planned to write on the role of the doctor in Latin America.

REMEMBERING ERNESTO,
A YOUNG DOCTOR IN MEXICO

A scientific research paper on allergies was presented by Dr. Ernesto Guevara de la Serna, then resident in Mexico City, and it was then published in Volume II, No.4 (May, 1955) of *Alergia: Revista Iberoamericana de Alergología*, edited by the late Dr. Mario Salazar Mallén, an eminent Mexican physician.

The newspaper and periodicals archive of the Medical Society of the General Hospital of Mexico, where the young doctor Ernesto Guevara practiced, preserves the originals of this and other research carried out by Ernesto. During that period, he worked both at the General Hospital and at the Institute of Cardiology, where Dr. Salazar Mallén led a research center.

What follows are excerpts from an interview conducted by journalist Marta Rojas, published in the Cuban newspaper *Granma*, June 14, 1989.

Mallén's widow, Olvido Tapia, recalls:

Professor Salazar Mallén was devoted to his profession and he wanted Ernesto Guevara to wholeheartedly devote himself to medicine just as he did, because he rightly believed that the kid had a great talent for research. My husband told me that ultimately he was unable to persuade him. Aware of his intentions, one day Ernesto confirmed his fears when he said, "Maestro... well, I'll see you around, I've made my decision." Later, when Mario learned of the *Granma* landing and the trials and tribulations that Fidel, Ernesto and all the others went through, he was furious, really furious that he had not been able to prevent Ernesto from leaving. He said to me, "You see, that kid is not going to last, remember his asthma." But life proved Che — as everyone called him — right, and not my husband. Then, in 1959, 1960, and so on, Che called Mario to consult him about medications and allergy problems. Mario also called him and informed him of how the research was going in that field; they remained great friends. Che invited him to Cuba to meet with doctors there, he took him to visit places where he had fought as a guerrilla with Commander Fidel Castro, and Mario brought many photographs back to Mexico in which Che, his bearded assistants, his wife Aleida March appeared...

He was so fond of Ernesto that he made him accompany us on excursions, almost all related to events on his medical specialty that were held in other states of the country. My daughter, then very little, and unfortunately also deceased, was very fond of Ernesto and he of her. He would pick her up and walk long distances carrying her on his back, simply to please her; he was very friendly and polite. When the professor was talking to other people that Ernesto did not know, he immediately separated from the group, and unless Mario called on him he didn't take part in the conversation, even when he mastered the subject in question perfectly. We even invited him as soon as he arrived to live in this house, where there was space and he would be comfortable, but Ernesto refused. He said that it was not right for a student to live in the same house as his professor, that the maestro needed privacy and that there were certain distances to be kept. There was no way of convincing him to come live with us. He preferred to be in a sleeping bag on an examination table in a small examination and instruments room in the hospital, until he could have his own apartment."

Dr. David Mitrani, a friend of Ernesto's in Mexico, remembers:

Che was just a year older than me. We were very young. I admired him. We all admired him at the hospital, because at the age of just 24 he had traveled all over Latin America. He had participated in the "uprising" in Guatemala... Anyway, as he was an Argentine, what he told us sometimes appeared to be an exaggeration, but it was the pure truth: he had lived life to the full then, and here in Mexico too. During the day he worked on his research, while at night he was an assistant lecturer in human physiology at the old School of Medicine. He also took photos. Meanwhile, he operated on dogs and cats for his research. The interesting thing was that he was very mature with such things, and at the same time he was like a big kid. For example, as Mrs. Olvido said, he played with little María Eugenia. The two of us discussed international politics a great deal; he was very mature.

[...]

The day after Ernesto met Fidel, he came to see me at the hospital. He was very excited, really enthusiastic, and told me that Fidel was a very likable and very intelligent person and several other things. Later, I got to know some Cubans whom I treated as a doctor in the hospital, at the express request of Ernesto. When he was taken prisoner he sent for me, he asked for adrenaline. I personally took some vials to him and the funny thing was that when I arrived at the jail, the first thing I came across with was Ernesto, Che, playing chess with one of the officers, with one of his jailers.

But returning to his interest in medicine, I can tell you that Ernesto worked very hard and very seriously, just as with everything he did. His research was successful. As a young man he had resounding success on having his work published in a specialized journal. I remember at least two very much talked-about papers on food antigens and the action of histamine in cats' uteri. He undertook the research alone and wrote the papers in the midst of his political concerns and the struggle to make a living, because he already had a family.

Ah, yes! At midday in the laboratory, the maestro (Salazar Mallén) had the habit of taking a break to drink coffee with us. During that time, a classic would be read, usually short stories by Mark Twain or Anton Chekhov. The maestro asked his students to comment on what had been read and Ernesto, with his maturity and culture, always offered enriching remarks. In the afternoon, when the work was finished in the laboratory, it was his moment: we invited girls and other colleagues and Che prepared two liters of *maté* tea, and we would talk, heatedly debate... Ernesto loved to prepare the *maté* and "forced" us to drink it with him, and we missed it when we no longer drank that *maté*. Then he and I would go out again to "*taquear*"[16] or to follow our respective individual interests.

---

[16]   To eat tacos on the street.

A GUERRILLA DOCTOR

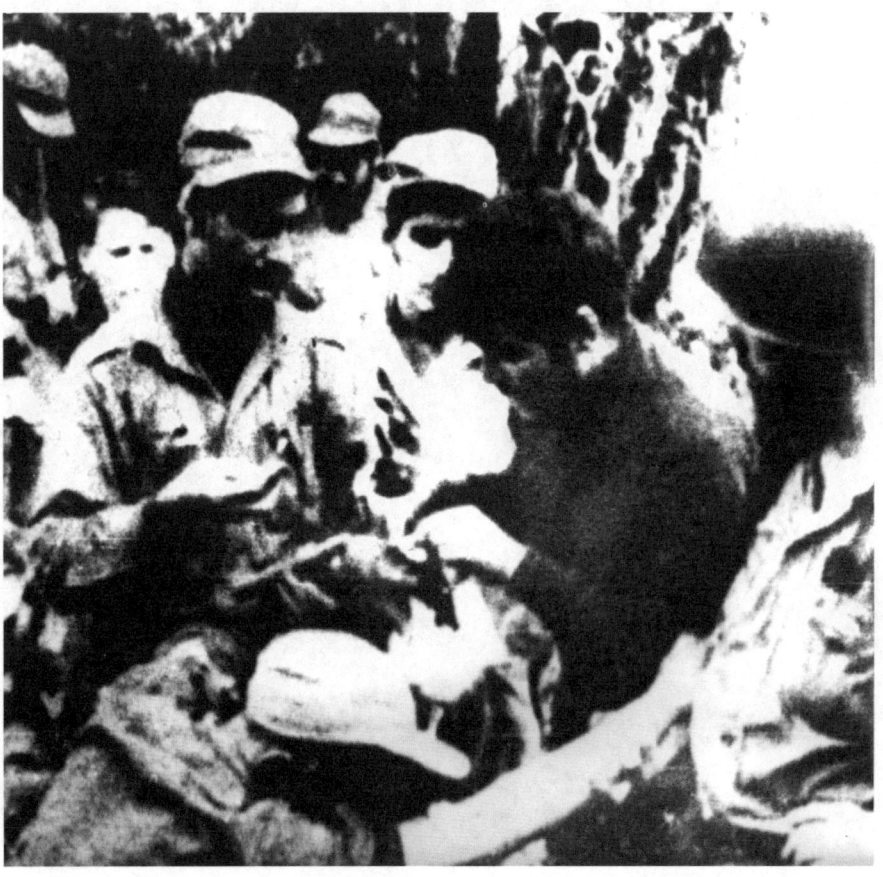

Che extracts a bullet from a wound in the Sierra Maestra.

REMINISCENCES
OF CUBA'S REVOLUTIONARY WAR

Excerpts from *Che's Reminiscences of the Cuban Revolutionary War.*

After the arrival in Cuba on the *Granma*, December 1956

All we had left of our equipment for war was nothing but our rifles, car-tridge belts, and a few wet rounds of ammunition. Our medical supplies had vanished, and most of our backpacks had been left behind in the swamps.

[…]

By daybreak on December 5 only a few could take another step. On the verge of collapse, we would walk a short distance and then beg for a long rest.

[…]

I was the troop physician and it was my duty to treat everyone's blistered feet. I recall my last patient that morning: his name was compañero Hum-berto Lamotte and it was to be his last day on earth. In my mind's eye I see how tired and anguished he was as he walked from my improvised first-aid station to his post, carrying in one hand the shoes he could not wear.

[…]

A compañero dropped a box of ammunition at my feet. I pointed to it, and he answered me with an anguished expression, which I remember per-fectly, and which seemed to say, "It's too late for ammunition." He imme-diately took the path to the cane field. (He was later murdered by Batista's henchmen.)

This might have been the first time I was faced, literally, with the dilemma of choosing between my devotion to medicine and my duty as a revolutio-nary soldier. There, at my feet, was a backpack full of medicine and a box of ammunition. They were too heavy to carry both. I picked up the ammunition, leaving the medicine, and started to cross the clearing, heading for the cane field.

[...]

Near me, a compañero named [Emilio] Albentosa was walking toward the cane field. A burst of gunfire hit us both. I felt a sharp blow to my chest and a wound in my neck; I thought for certain I was dead. Albentosa, vomiting blood and bleeding profusely from a deep wound made by a .45-caliber bullet, screamed something like, "They've killed me," and began to fire his rifle although there was no one there. Flat on the ground, I said to Faustino, "I'm fucked," and Faustino, still shooting, looked at me and told me it was nothing, but I saw in his eyes he considered me as good as dead.

[...]

Almeida approached, urging me to go on, and despite the intense pain I dragged myself into the cane field. There I saw the great compañero Raúl Suárez, whose thumb had been blown away by a bullet, being attended by Faustino Pérez, who was bandaging his hand. *("Alegría de Pío.")*

Doing things differently
January 1957

Our attitude toward the wounded was in stark contrast to that of Batista's army. Not only did they kill our wounded men, they abandoned their own. Over time this difference had an effect on the enemy and it was a factor in our victory. Fidel ordered that the prisoners be given all available medicine to take care of the wounded. This decision pained me because, as a doctor, I felt the need to save all available medicine for our own troops. *("The Battle of La Plata.")*

"You Argentine son of a…"
February–March 1957

Everybody was able to reach the peak easily, and pass over it; but for me it was a tremendous effort. I made it to the top, but with such an asthma attack that each step was difficult. I remember how much work Crespo put in to help me when I could not go on and pleaded they leave me behind. The *guajiro*, in that particular language among the troops, said to me, "You Argentine son of a…! You'll walk or I'll hit you with my rifle butt." With everything he was already carrying, he virtually carried both me and my pack, as we made it over the hill with a heavy downpour against our backs. (*"Bitter Days."*)

General Staff physician
March 1957

The new platoons were also organized, integrating the entire troop and forming three groups under the direction of captains Raúl Castro, Juan Almeida, and Jorge Sotús; Camilo Cienfuegos would lead the forward guard and Efigenio Ameijeiras the rear guard; I was general staff physician and Universo Sánchez functioned as general staff squadron leader. (*"Reinforcements."*)

Tempering the troops
March–April 1957

I was assigned a new recruit, Paulino [Fonseca], as an assistant to carry the medical supplies. This eased my burden a little so that for a few minutes each day after our long marches I could attend to our troop's health. (*"Tempering the Troops."*)

"That doctor tells everyone the same thing"
May 1957

In that period I was still working as a doctor and in each little village or hamlet I set up a consultation area. It was monotonous, for I had little medicine to offer and the clinical cases in the Sierra Maestra were all more or less the same: prematurely aged and toothless women, children with distended bellies, parasites, rickets, general vitamin deficiencies — these were the stains of the Sierra Maestra.

[...]

I remember one girl was watching the consultations I was giving to the local women, who came in with an almost religious attitude toward finding the sources of their sufferings. When her mother arrived, the little girl — after attentively watching several previous examinations in the hut that served as a clinic — gaily remarked, "Mamá, that doctor says the same thing to everyone!"

And it was absolutely true; my knowledge was good for little else. They all had the same clinical symptoms, and without knowing it they each told the same heartbreaking story. What would have happened if the doctor had diagnosed the strange exhaustion suffered by the young mother of several children, when she carried buckets of water from the river to the house, as being simply due to too much work on such a meager diet? Her exhaustion is inexplicable to her, since all her life she had carried the same buckets of water to the same place and only now does she feel tired.

[...]

I only know that for me, those consultations with the peasants of the Sierra Maestra converted my spontaneous and somewhat lyrical resolve into a different, more serene force. Those suffering and loyal inhabitants of the Sierra Maestra have never suspected the role they played in forging our revolutionary ideology. (*"On the March."*)

A full-time combatant
May 1957

One of the machine guns went to Captain Jorge Sotús's platoon, another to Almeida's, and the third to the general staff, for which I had responsibility. The tripods were distributed as follows: one for Raúl, another for Guillermo García, and the third for Crescencio Pérez. In this way, I began as a full-time combatant, for until then I had been the troop's doctor, only participating in occasional combat. I had entered a new stage. (*"The Weapons Arrive."*)

The Battle of El Uvero
May 1957

Near me I heard a groan and then some shouts amid the din of battle. I thought it must be a wounded enemy soldier, and I dragged myself forward, shouting for him to surrender. But it was compañero Leal, wounded in the head. I examined him quickly and found both entrance and exit wounds were in the parietal region. Leal was losing consciousness, and the limbs on one side of his body — I don't remember which — were becoming paralyzed. The only bandage I had on hand was a piece of paper that I placed over the wounds.

[...]

We reached the warehouse and took prisoner the two soldiers who had escaped my shots, as well as the post doctor and his assistant. The doctor was a quiet, gray-haired man whose subsequent fate I am unaware of; I don't know whether he joined the revolution. A curious thing happened with this man: my medical knowledge has never been that great, the number of wounded was enormous, and my vocation at that moment was not focused on health. When I brought the wounded to the military doctor, he asked me how old I was and when I had finished my training. I explained that it had been some years ago, and he said frankly, "Look, son, you'd better take charge of all this because I've just graduated and I have very little experience." Between his lack of experience and his natural fear on finding himself prisoner, he had forgotten every medical fact he ever knew. So once again I had to swap my rifle for a doctor's coat, which really involved little more than a wash of my hands.

[...]

My return to the medical profession was quite emotional. The first patient I attended, the most gravely wounded, was compañero Cilleros. A bullet had split open his right arm and, after piercing a lung, had apparently embedded itself in his spine, paralyzing both legs. His condition was critical, and I was only able to give him a sedative and bind his chest tightly so he could breathe more easily. We tried to save him in the only way possible: we took the 14 prisoners with us and left the two wounded guerrillas, Leal and Cilleros, with the enemy, on the doctor's word of honor that they would be cared for. When I told this to Cilleros, mouthing the usual words of comfort, he answered with a sad smile that, more than any words could have, expressed his conviction that it was all over. We knew this as well, and I was tempted at that moment to place a farewell kiss on his forehead. Yet, coming from me, more than anyone else, such an act would have signified a death sentence for our compañero, and duty told me that I must not make his last minutes more bitter with the confirmation of something he already knew. I said goodbye, as sweetly as possible and with enormous pain, to the two combatants who remained in the hands of the enemy. They proclaimed that they would prefer to die among their compañeros; but we also had the duty to fight to the end for their lives. So there they remained, brothers now with 19 wounded Batista soldiers whom we had treated as best we could. Our two compañeros were decently treated by the enemy army, but Cilleros did not make it to Santiago. Leal survived his wound, was imprisoned on the Isle of Pines for the rest of the war, and today still bears the indelible scars of that important episode in our revolutionary war.

[…]

In one of Babún's trucks we hauled the largest possible quantity of every kind of equipment, especially medical. We left last, heading toward our mountain hideout, which we reached in time to care for the wounded and take leave of the dead, who were buried at a bend in the road.

We realized there would now be an intense pursuit and decided that those men who could walk should move away quickly, leaving the wounded behind in my care. Enrique López was to furnish me with transport, a hiding place, some assistants to help move the wounded, and the necessary contacts through which we could receive medicines and properly treat the men. (*"The Battle of Uvero."*)

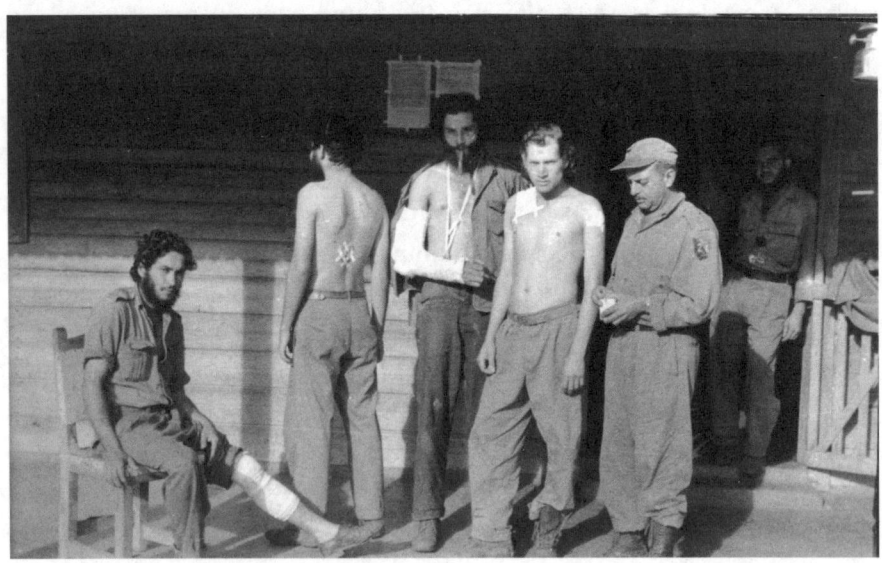

Field hospital in Las Villas.

The situation was difficult
May–June 1957

Almeida and Pena could not walk; neither could Quike Escalona. I recommended Manals not walk either because of the wound in his lung. Manuel Acuña, Hermes Leyva, and Maceo could all walk on their own. To defend, nurse, and transport them, there were Vilo Acuña, the guide Sinecio Torres, Joel Iglesias, Alejandro Oñate, and myself.

[...]

The situation was difficult. Quike Escalona's wounds were infected and I could not determine the gravity of Manals's injuries. We explored the nearby roads without encountering enemy soldiers, and decided to move the wounded to a peasant hut three or four kilometers away. The owner had abandoned it, leaving behind a good number of chickens.

[...]

With our few available men we started on a short but very difficult trek down to Indio Creek. We then climbed a narrow path to a small shack where a peasant named Israel lived with his wife and brother-in-law. Moving our wounded compañeros through such rugged terrain was grueling work, but we did it, and the two peasants even gave us their own double bed for the wounded to sleep in.

[...]

After a short time, Acuña and Joel Iglesias told me they had heard strange voices on the other slope. We honestly believed the hour had come when we would be forced to fight under the most difficult circumstances. It was our obligation to defend to the death the precious cargo of wounded men we had been entrusted with.

[...]

The following day, six months after the landing of the *Granma*, we began our march early. These treks were tiring, and incredibly short for anyone accustomed to long marches in the mountains. We could carry only one wounded compañero at a time, and we had to carry them in hammocks hanging from strong branches that literally ruined the shoulders of the bearers. Bearers had to relieve each other every 10 or 15 minutes, so that we needed six or eight to carry each wounded man. (*"Caring for the Wounded."*)

I debut as a dentist
June 1957

We spent the whole month of June 1957 nursing our compañeros wounded in the battle of El Uvero, and organizing our small troop, which would return to Fidel's column.

[...]

My asthma was somewhat aggravated and the lack of medicine meant I was almost as immobile as the wounded. I was able to relieve the illness somewhat by smoking dried clarín flowers, a local remedy, until medicine arrived from civilization. This helped me to restore my health in preparation for our leaving, but day after day, our departure was delayed.

[...]

On June 26, I debuted as dentist, although in the Sierra Maestra I was given the more modest title of "tooth-puller." My first victim was Israel Pardo, today a captain in the army, who came out of it pretty well. The second was Joel Iglesias, who would have needed a stick of dynamite to remove his canine tooth; in fact, he saw out the end of the war with the tooth still in place since my efforts to extract it had been fruitless. Besides the meagerness of my skill, we had no anesthetic, so I frequently used "psychological anesthesia" — a few harsh epithets when my patients complained too much about what was going on in their mouths.

[...]

After short, arduous marches, we reached the region of Palma Mocha, on the western slope of Turquino, near Las Cuevas. The peasants received us very well and we established direct contact through my new profession as "tooth-puller," which I exercised with great enthusiasm. *("Return Journey.")*

A new doctor joins the guerrilla forces
July 1957

At the last meeting we met a new doctor who had joined the guerrilla forces: Sergio del Valle [...]

("Betrayal in the Making.")

"Don't kill me, don't kill me!"
August 1957

A few reconnaissance planes flew high over us and, just to be safe, we stopped in a store and attended to the three wounded men. One had a slight wound in the shoulder but it had torn the flesh, so treatment was somewhat difficult. One had a slight wound in the hand from a small-caliber weapon. The third had a bump on his head: when the mules in the barracks, frightened or wounded by the shooting, had begun to kick wildly, they had apparently dislodged some plaster that had fallen on his head. *("The Attack on Bueycito.")*

Pino del Agua
September 1957

Every time one of our combatants passed near [a wounded soldier] he would shout, "Don't kill me! Don't kill me! Che says not to kill prisoners!" When the battle was over, we transported him to the sawmill and gave him first aid. *("Pino del Agua.")*

Extracting a bullet with a razor
December 1957

A day or two after the battle, Machadito [José Ramón Machado], today the minister of public health, operated on me with a razor, extracting an M-1 bullet. From then on, my recovery was rapid.

("Altos de Conrado.")

Organizing hospitals
December 1957

As for medicines, we obtained them in the cities, not always in the quantity or quality we needed; but at least we were able to maintain some kind of functioning apparatus for their acquisition.

[...]

Concerning the organization the life in the camps and communications, certain sanitary regulations were established, and in this period the first hospitals were organized. One was set up in the zone under my command, in an inaccessible place that offered relative security to the wounded, since it was invisible from the air. But it was in the heart of a dense woods, and dampness made it unhealthy for the wounded and sick. This hospital was organized by compañero Sergio del Valle. The doctors Martínez Páez, Vallejo, and Piti Fajardo organized similar hospitals in Fidel's column, but these were only improved during the second year of the struggle. *("One Year of Armed Struggle.")*

"Don't worry, commander, I will die with you"
April 1958

My asthma, mercifully, had let me run a few meters, but it was taking its revenge and my heart was jumping inside my chest. I heard branches breaking as someone approached, but it was no longer possible to keep fleeing (which was what I really felt like doing). This time, it was another compañero, lost: a recruit who had recently joined our troop. His consolation was more or less, "Don't worry, commander, I will die with you." *("Interlude.")*

...and I earned it here
May–December 1958

In Santa Clara, while speaking to the wounded in the Sangre Hospital, a dying man touched my hand and said, "Remember, commander? In Remedios you sent me to find a weapon… and I earned it here." He was the combatant who had accidentally fired his weapon. He died a few minutes later, I think content for having proven his courage. Such was our Rebel Army. *("The Final Offensive and the Battle of Santa Clara.")*

GUERRILLA WARFARE

Excerpts from *Che's Guerrilla Warfare.*

The guerrilla fighter as combatant

A wounded enemy should be treated with care and respect unless his former life warrants the death penalty, in which case he will be treated according to his deserts.

[…]

The guerrilla fighter must never for any reason leave a wounded compañero at the mercy of the enemy troops, because this means abandoning them to an almost certain death. At whatever cost, the wounded must be removed from the combat zone to a secure place. The greatest exertions and the greatest risks must be taken in this task. The guerrilla soldier must be an extraordinary compañero.

Health

One of the serious problems a guerrilla fighter confronts is exposure to the accidents of life, especially to wounds and illness, which are very common in guerrilla warfare. The doctor performs an extraordinarily important role in the guerrilla band, not just in saving lives, where their scientific intervention might have little impact because of the limited resources available; the doctor also reinforces the patient's morale and makes them feel that there is someone nearby who is dedicating their entire effort to minimizing their pain; the doctor gives the sick or wounded the comfort of knowing that someone will remain at their side until they are cured or out of danger.

The organization of hospitals depends largely on the stage of development of the guerrilla band. Three fundamental types of hospital organization corresponding to various stages can be mentioned.

In the first, nomadic phase, the doctor — if there is one — always travels with their compañeros, as just one more person; they will probably have to perform all the other functions of the guerrilla fighter, including that of fighting, and will suffer at times the depressing and desperate task of treating patients when the means of saving lives are not available. This is the stage in which the doctor has the most influence over the troops, the greatest impact on their morale. During this period of the guerrilla band's development the doctor achieves their full potential as a true priest, who seems to carry in their poorly equipped backpack the consolation needed by the guerrillas. The value of a simple aspirin to someone who is suffering badly is beyond calculation, when administered by the friendly hand of someone who makes that suffering his own. Therefore, in the first stage, the doctor must be a person who totally identifies with the ideas of the revolution, because their words will affect the troops much more deeply than those of any other member.

In the normal course of events in guerrilla warfare a further stage is reached that might be called "semi-nomadic." There will be camps, occasionally visited by the guerrilla troops; friendly, secure houses where it is possible to store objects and even leave the wounded; and a growing tendency for the guerrilla troop to become settled. At this stage, the task of the doctor is less frustrating; they might have emergency surgical equipment in their backpack and another more complete kit for less urgent operations in a friendly house. It will be possible to leave the sick and wounded in the care of peasants who will offer their help with great dedication. The doctor can also count on a greater number of medicines kept in convenient places; as far as possible, these should be completely catalogued, depending on the circumstances. In this same semi-nomadic state, if the guerrilla band operates in places that are absolutely inaccessible, hospitals can be established to which the sick and wounded can go to recover.

In the third stage, when there are zones invulnerable to the enemy, a true hospital network can be constructed. In its most developed form, this might consist of three different types of center. In the combat category there should be a doctor, the combatant most loved by the troops, a fighter, who does not need very extensive knowledge. I say this because their task is principally one of giving relief and preparing the sick or wounded, while the real medical work is performed in hospitals situated more securely. A good surgeon should not be sacrificed in the line of fire.

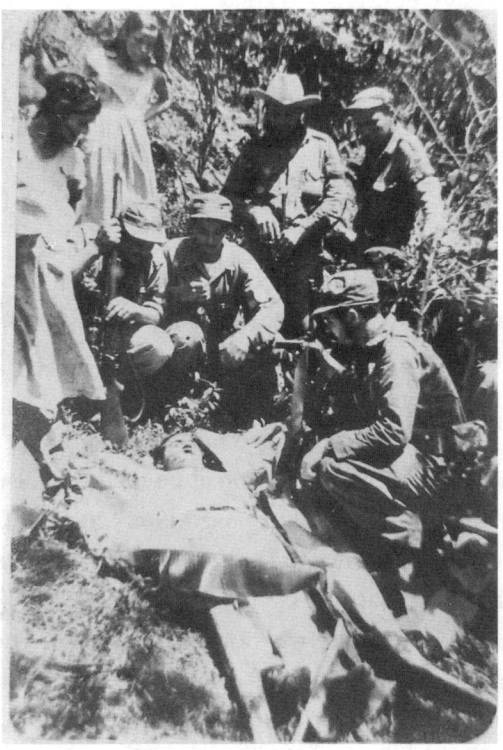

When soldiers fall in the front line, stretcher-bearers — if available, which will depend on the level of organization of the guerrilla band — will carry the wounded to the first post; if they are not available, the compañeros themselves will perform this duty. Transport of the wounded in rough zones is one of the most delicate of all tasks and one of the most painful experiences in a soldier's life. The transport of the wounded is probably harder on the compañeros than the wounded soldier, however grave the injury, because of the guerrillas' spirit of sacrifice. The transport can be carried out in different ways depending on the nature of the terrain. In rough and wooded places, which are typical in this kind of warfare, it is necessary to walk in single file. Here the best system is to use a long pole, with the patient carried in a hammock that hangs from it.

The guerrillas take turns carrying the weight, one in front and one behind. They should swap positions with two other compañeros frequently, since the shoulders suffer severely and the individual is gradually worn out carrying this delicate and heavy burden.

After having been checked at the first hospital, the wounded soldier then proceeds with the information of this initial treatment to a second center, where there might be surgeons and specialists, depending on the possibilities of the guerrilla troop, and where more serious life-saving operations are performed and individuals can be relieved from danger — this is the second stage.

At a third level, there are much better hospitals that can conduct investigations into causes and effects of illnesses that prevail among the residents of the zone. These hospitals, which correspond to a sedentary life, are not only centers for convalescence and for less urgent operations, but also serve the civil population, where the hygiene specialists have an educational role. Dispensaries that can monitor individual treatment should also be established. If the supply capability of the civil organization is sufficient, the hospitals of this third group can have a range of facilities that provide diagnosis, possibly even laboratory and x-ray facilities.

Other useful individuals are the doctor's assistants. They are generally youths with some vocation and some knowledge, with fairly strong physiques; they do not bear arms, sometimes because their vocation is medicine, but usually because there are insufficient arms for everyone who wants them. These assistants will be in charge of carrying most of the medicines, an extra stretcher, or a hammock, if circumstances make this possible. They must take charge of the wounded in any battle that is fought.

The essential medicines should be obtained through contacts with health organizations that exist in the enemy's territory. Sometimes they can be obtained from such organizations as the International Red Cross, but this should not be counted on, especially in the initial period of the struggle. It is necessary to organize an apparatus that will ensure the rapid transport of the medicines required in case of danger and that will gradually provide all the hospitals with the supplies necessary for their work, military as well as civil. Moreover, contacts should be made in the surrounding areas with doctors who would be able to help the wounded whose cases are beyond the capacities or the facilities of the guerrilla band.

The doctors required for this type of warfare have different characteristics. The combatant doctor, the compañero of the guerrillas, is needed in the first stage; their functions develop as the action of the guerrilla band becomes more complicated and a range of connected organizations is created. General surgeons are the best acquisition for an army of this type. If an anesthetist is available, so much the better; although almost all operations are performed not with gas anesthesia but using largactil and sodium pentothal, which are much easier to administer and easier to procure and preserve. Besides general surgeons, bone specialists are very useful, because fractures often occur from accidents in the zone; they are also often the result of bullet wounds in limbs. The clinic primarily serves the peasant masses, since sicknesses in the guerrilla armies are generally easy for anyone to diagnose. The most difficult task is to cure problems caused by nutritional deficiencies.

In a more advanced stage, if there are good hospitals, there might even be laboratory technicians, in order to have complete facilities. Appeals should be made to all sectors of the profession whose services are needed; it is quite likely that many will respond to this call and come to offer their help. All kinds of medical professionals are needed; surgeons are very useful, so are dentists. Dentists should be advised to come with simple field instruments and a campaign-type drill, with which they can do practically everything necessary.

CHE AS A LEADER OF THE CUBAN REVOLUTION

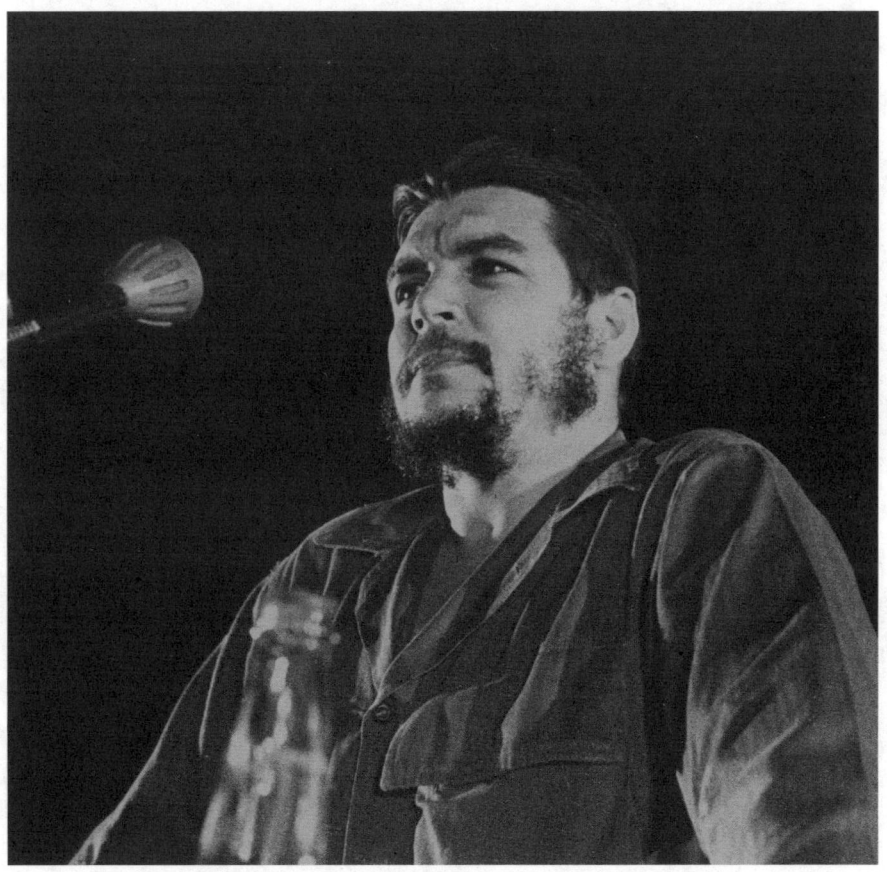

Speech on the steps of the University of Havana, November 27, 1961,
to commemorate the anniversary of the 1871 execution of medical students
by Spanish colonial authorities.

AT THE MEDICAL ASSOCIATION

Speech at a ceremony held in Che's honor, organized by the Cuban Medical Association
January 16, 1959.

The truth is that I do not come here with any concealed discourse, like someone who shows up with a speech under his arm, declining the undeserved honor of being chosen to speak because he is not prepared. I came here to fulfill my somewhat forgotten duties as a doctor to present my greetings, nothing more.

Frankly, I am somewhat unaccustomed, or rather, I am totally unaccustomed to occupying the chair or the platform of a meeting of professionals, and I believe that if my life had followed the path of science, I would never have arrived here. This shows that the big shots still have their belligerence in the Americas, as I was so easily able to come here to this platform and say a few words.

Just to say that I believe no one should be surprised in any way that a foreigner should come to fight for Cuba, because it was precisely in Cuba that [José] Martí lived, spoke and taught, whose greatest aspiration was to unite all Latin America. I confess that I have never felt like a foreigner, neither in Cuba nor in any of the countries I have traveled through in my somewhat adventurous life. I felt Guatemalan in Guatemala, Mexican in Mexico, Peruvian in Peru, just as I feel Cuban today in Cuba. And naturally, I likewise feel Argentine here and everywhere. That is the essence of my personality; I cannot forget the *mate* and the *asado*.

I believe, since we are here, that we could talk about something even more important: the necessary contribution of the medical class to our revolution, not as regards what it has already given, because what it has already contributed is recognized by everyone. Of all the professions, the medical profession has perhaps been the one that has sacrificed the most blood, the most men to the revolution. I do not remember any of our columns that did not include the services of a doctor and sometimes more than one.

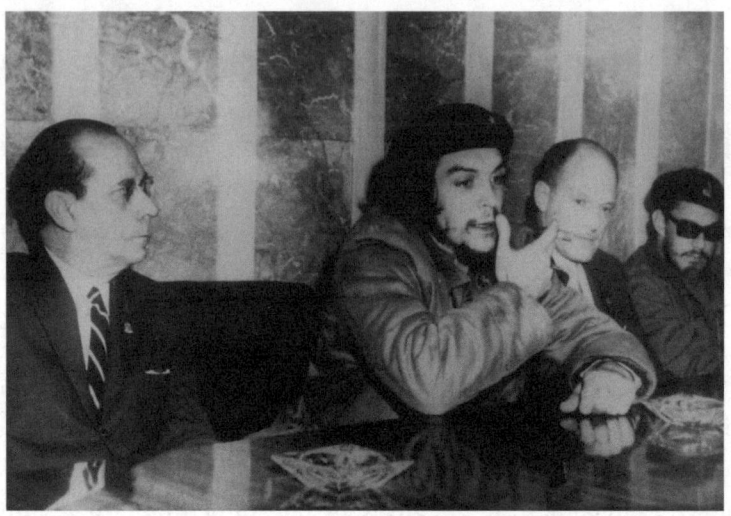

At the Cuban Medical Association, 1959.

As a doctor who has always been concerned about social issues, I believe that now is the time to make a substantial contribution to radically change the prevailing health system in Cuba, as in all nations.

In this somewhat curious journey I made through all the countries of Latin America, I unfortunately noted that one of the things that was most backward was health care, and our experience in the Sierra Maestra was that there is no health care there.

Many young people in Mexico told me that Cuba was different, that Cuba was not a country like Mexico, where there is zero health care outside the capital. But I have realized that in many parts of Cuba health care is also completely unknown.

The Sierra Maestra is a place in Cuba that seemed like somewhere far from Cuba, to be somewhere else entirely. Later on, I saw a completely different situation in the cities and also in the richest agricultural areas and the countryside.

I believe that what we have to do now, in these days of triumph and peace, is to prepare ourselves to fight honestly and fervently for the entire

Cuban health system to take an important step forward, to be able to build all the clinics and services in those neglected areas and also to modernize many others.

We have not yet had the opportunity to visit research centers and many services here in the capital, but I realize that there is still much to be done. And I take the liberty of initiating some criticism here, precisely because I consider myself Cuban and I believe that I not only have the right but the duty to draw attention to anything I find wrong.

I believe that now is the time to start thinking seriously, as I was commenting a moment ago to my compañeros Dr. del Valle and Dr. Rodríguez, about the new direction that medicine must take in Cuba. We have made a revolution that is perhaps absolutely historic and marks a new step in the development of the peoples of the Americas' struggle for their liberation. Thus, we must also complete this struggle and revolution in all branches and bravely take social medicine forward as far as possible.

Of course, I am not going to set any guidelines now because I do not have the training to do so. I merely call attention to this point. Besides, it is also my turn now to apologize for getting in over my head and talking about things that I should not mention. In any case, here I should have spoken about guerrilla issues, which I know well because I have learned them, and not about medical issues. But since I have been invited by the Medical Association and I was given the opportunity to say a few words, I wanted to call the attention of all my compañeros to this matter.

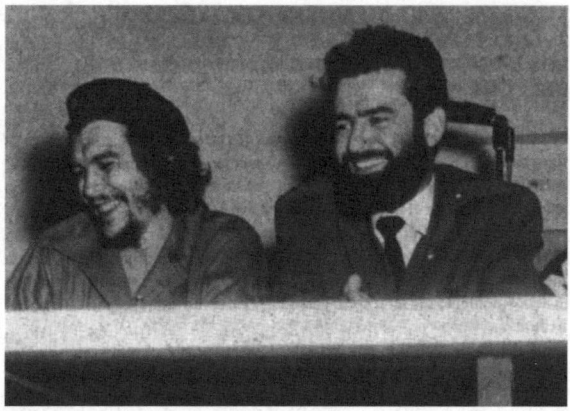

At the Medical Association alongside Dr. Oscar Fernández Mell.

ON REVOLUTIONARY MEDICINE

Speech given at the inauguration of a training course at the Ministry of Public Health on August 19, 1960.

Compañeros:

Although this modest ceremony is only one among hundreds held as the of Cuban people celebrate day by day their freedom and the advance of all their revolutionary laws, their advance along the road to total independence, I nevertheless find it interesting.

Almost everyone knows that I started my career as a doctor some years ago. And when I started off as a doctor, when I began to study medicine, the majority of the concepts I hold today as a revolutionary were absent from the storehouse of my ideals.

I wanted to succeed, as everybody wants to succeed. I dreamed about being a famous researcher. I dreamed of working tirelessly to achieve something that could really be put at the disposal of humanity, but that, at the same time, would be a personal triumph. I was, as we all are, a child of my environment.

Through particular circumstances, and perhaps also because of my character, after receiving my degree I set out to travel through Latin America and I got to know it intimately. Except for Haiti and the Dominican Republic, I have visited — in one way of another — all the other countries of Latin America. And in the way I traveled, first as a student and afterward as a doctor, I began to come into close contact with poverty, with hunger, with disease, with the inability to cure a child because of lack of resources, with the numbness that hunger and continued deprivation cause until a point is reached where a parent losing a child is an unimportant accident, as often happens among the embattled classes of our Latin American homeland. And I began to see that there was something that, at that time, seemed to me almost as important as being a famous researcher or making some substantial contribution to medical science, and that was helping those people.

But I continued being, as all of us always continue being, a child of my environment, and I wanted to help those people through my personal efforts. I had already traveled a lot — I was then in Guatemala, the Guatemala of Arbenz — and I had begun to make some notes to guide the conduct of a revolutionary doctor. I began to look into what I needed to be a revolutionary doctor.

However, the aggression came [in Guatemala], aggression unleashed by the United Fruit Company, the State Department, Foster Dulles — in reality, they're all the same thing — and the puppet they put in named Castillo Armas — that was his name. The aggression was successful, given that the people had not yet reached the level of [political] maturity the Cuban people have today. And one fine day, I, like so many others, took the road to exile, or at least I took the road of fleeing from Guatemala, since it was not my homeland.

Then I realized one fundamental thing: to be a revolutionary doctor or to be a revolutionary, there must first be a revolution. The isolated effort, the individual effort, the purity of ideals, the desire to sacrifice an entire lifetime to the noblest of ideals goes for naught if that effort is made alone, solitary, in some corner of Latin America, fighting against hostile governments and social conditions that do not permit progress. A revolution needs what we have in Cuba: an entire people mobilized, who have learned the use of arms and the practice of combative unity, who know what a weapon is worth and what the people's unity is worth.

And then we get to the heart of the problem that today lies ahead of us. We already have the right and even the obligation to be, before anything else, a revolutionary doctor, that is, a person who puts the technical knowledge of his profession at the service of the revolution and of the people. Then we come back to the earlier questions: How does one do a job of social welfare effectively? How does one reconcile individual effort with the needs of society?

We again have to recall what each of our lives was like, what each of us did and thought, as a doctor or in any other public health function, prior to the revolution. We have to do so with profound critical enthusiasm. And we will then conclude that almost everything we thought and felt in that past epoch should be filed away, and that a new type of human being should be created. And if each one of us is their own architect of that new human type, then creating that new type of human being — who will be the representative of the new Cuba — will be much easier.

It is good for you — those present, the residents of Havana — to absorb this idea: that in Cuba a new type of human being is being created, which cannot be entirely appreciated in the capital, but which can be seen in every corner of the country. Those of you who went to the Sierra Maestra on July 26 must have seen two absolutely unheard-of things: an army with picks and shovels, an army that takes the greatest pride in marching in the patriotic celebrations in Oriente Province with its picks and shovels ready, while the militia compañeros are marching with their rifles. But you must have also seen something much more important: You must have seen some children who by their physical stature appear eight or nine years old, but who nevertheless are almost all thirteen or fourteen. They are the most authentic children of the Sierra Maestra, the most authentic children of hunger and poverty in all its forms. They are the creatures of malnutrition.

In this small Cuba, with four or five television channels, with hundreds of radio stations, with all the advances of modern science, when those children arrived at school at night for the first time and saw the electric lights, they exclaimed that the stars were very low that night. Those children, whom some of you would have seen, are now learning in the collective schools, from the ABCs right up to learning a trade, right up to the very difficult science of being revolutionaries.

These are the new types of human beings born in Cuba. They are being born in isolated places, in remote points in the Sierra Maestra and also in the cooperatives and centers of work.

All that has a lot to do with the topic of our talk today: the integration of the doctor and every other medical worker into the revolutionary movement. Because the revolution's task — the task of training and nourishing the children, the task of educating the army, the task of distributing the lands of the old absentee landlords among those who sweated every day on that same land without reaping its fruit — is the greatest work of social medicine that has been done in Cuba.

The battle against disease should be based on the principle of creating a robust body — not creating a robust body through a doctor's artistic work on a weak organism, but creating a robust body through the world of the whole collectivity, especially the whole social collectivity.

One day medicine will have to become a science that serves to prevent diseases, to orient the entire public toward their medical obligations, and that intervention is only necessary in cases of extreme urgency to perform some surgical operation or to deal with something uncharacteristic of that new society we are creating.

The work that is today entrusted to the Ministry of Health, to all the institutions of this type, is to organize public health in such a manner that it aids the greatest possible number of people, that it prevents everything foreseeable related to diseases, and that it orients the people. But for the organizational task, as for all revolutionary tasks, what is required, fundamentally, is the individual. The revolution is not, as some claim, a standardizer of collective will, of collective initiative. To the contrary, it is a liberator of an individual's capacity.

What the revolution does do, however, is to orient that capacity. And our task today is to orient the creative talent of all the medical professionals toward the tasks of social medicine.

We are at the end of an era, and not only here in Cuba. Despite all that is said to the contrary and despite all the hopes of some people, the forms of capitalism we have known, under which we have been raised and have suffered, are being defeated throughout the world.

The monopolies are being defeated. Collective science every day registers new and important triumphs. And we have had the pride and the self-sacrificing duty of being the vanguard in Latin America of a liberation movement that began some time ago, in the other subjugated continents of Africa and Asia. And that very profound social change also demands very profound changes in the mentality of the people.

Individualism as such, as the isolated action of a person alone in a social environment, must disappear in Cuba. Individualism tomorrow should be the proper utilization of the whole person to the absolute benefit of the community. But even when all this is understood today, even when these things I am saying are comprehended, and even when everyone is willing to think a little about the present, about the past, and about what the future should be, changing the manner of thinking requires profound internal changes and helping bring about profound external changes, primarily social.

And those external changes are taking place in Cuba every day. One way of learning about this revolution, of getting to know the forces the people have within, forces that have been dormant for so long, is to visit every part of Cuba, visit the cooperatives and all the work centers being created. And one way of getting to the heart of the medical question is not only knowing, not only visiting these places, but also getting to know the people who make up these cooperatives and work centers. Go there and find out what diseases they have, what their ailments are, what extreme poverty they have lived in over the years, inherited from centuries of repression and total submission. The doctor, the medical worker, should then go to the heart of this new work, which is as a person among the masses, someone within the community.

Whatever happens in the world, by always being close to the patient, by knowing their psychology so deeply, by being the representative of those who come near pain and relieve it, the doctor always has a very important job, a job of great responsibility in social life.

Only a few months ago, it so happened here in Havana that a group of students, recently certified as doctors, did not want to go to the countryside and were demanding extra payment for going. From the viewpoint of the past it is most logical that this would occur; at least it seems that way to me, and I understand it perfectly. I simply remember that this was the way it was, the way it was regarded some years ago. Once more it is the gladiator in rebellion, the solitary fighter who wants to ensure a better future, better conditions, and to achieve recognition of the necessity of what he does.

But what would happen if it were not those kids — the majority of whose families could afford several years of study — who completed their courses and are now beginning to practice their profession? What if instead it was 200 or 300 peasants who had emerged, let's say by magic, from the university lecture halls?

What would have happened, simply, is that those peasants would have run immediately, and with great enthusiasm, to attend to their brothers and sisters. They would have requested posts with the most responsibility and the most work, in order to show that the years of study given them were not in vain. What would have happened is what will happen within six or seven years, when the new students, children of the working class and the peasantry, receive their professional degrees of whatever type.

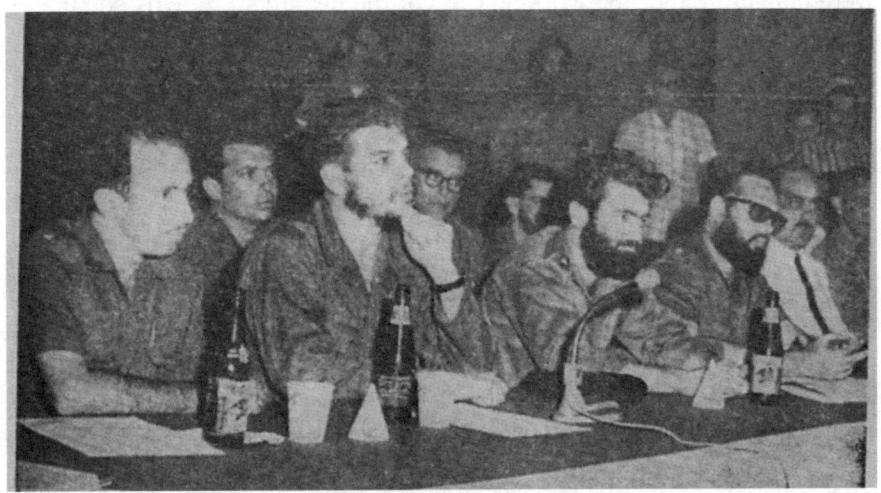

At the Ministry of Public Health, August 19, 1960.

But we should not view the future with fatalism and divide people into children of the working class or peasantry and counterrevolutionaries. Because that is simplistic, because it is not true, and because there is nothing that educates an honorable person more than living within a revolution.

Because none of us, none of the first group that arrived in the *Granma*, who established ourselves in the Sierra Maestra, and who learned to respect the peasant and the worker, living together with them — none of us had had a past as a worker or peasant. Naturally, there were those who had to work, who had known certain wants in their childhood. But hunger, true hunger — that none of us had known, and we began to know it — temporarily — during the two long years in the Sierra Maestra. And then many things became very clear.

We, who at the beginning severely punished anyone who touched even an egg of some rich peasant or some landowner, one day took 10,000 head of cattle to the Sierra and told the peasants simply: "Eat." And the peasants, for the first time in many years, and some for the first time in their lives, ate beef.

And the respect we had for the sacrosanct property of those 10,000 head of cattle was lost in the course of the armed struggle, and we understood perfectly that the life of a single human being is worth a million times more than all the property of the richest man on earth. And we learned it there, we who were not children of the working class or the peasantry. So why should we now shout to the four winds that we are the privileged ones and that the rest of the Cuban people cannot learn too? Yes, they can learn. In fact, the revolution today demands that they learn, demands that they understand well that the pride of serving our fellow human beings is much more important than a good income; that the people's gratitude is much more permanent, much more lasting than all the gold one can accumulate. And each doctor, in the sphere of their activity, can and should accumulate that prized treasure, the people's gratitude.

We must then begin to erase our old concepts and come even closer and ever more critically to the people. Not in the way we got closer before, because all of you will say: "No, I am a friend of the people. I enjoy talking with workers and peasants, and on Sundays I go to such and such a place to see such and such a thing." Everybody has done that. But they have done it practicing charity, and what we have to practice today is solidarity. We should not draw closer to the people to say: "Here we are. We come to give you the charity of our presence, to teach you with our science, to demonstrate your errors, your lack of refinement, your lack of elementary knowledge." We should go with an investigative zeal and with a humble spirit, to learn from the great source of wisdom that is the people.

Often we realize how mistaken we were in concepts we knew so well; they had become part of us and, automatically, of our consciousness. Every so often we ought to change all our ideas, not just general, social or philosophical concepts, but also, at times, our medical concepts. We will see that diseases are not always treated as one treats an illness in a big-city hospital. We will see then that the doctor also has to be a farmer, that one has to learn to cultivate new foods and, by their example, to cultivate the desire to consume new foods, to diversify this food structure in Cuba — so small and so poor in an agricultural country that is potentially the richest on earth. We will then see that under those circumstances we will have to be a little bit pedagogic, at times very pedagogic, that we will also have to be politic; that the first thing we will have to do is not go offering our wisdom, but showing that we are ready to learn with the people, to carry out that great and beautiful common experience — to build a new Cuba.

We have already taken many steps, and the distance between that January 1, 1959, and today cannot be measured in the conventional manner. It was some time ago that the people understood that not only had a dictator fallen here, but that a system had fallen as well. Now the people should learn that upon the ruins of a crumbled system, one must build a new one that brings about the people's absolute happiness.

I remember when Compañero [Nicolás] Guillén arrived from Argentina early last year. He was the same great poet he is today — perhaps his books were translated into one fewer language, because every day he wins new readers in all the languages of the world — but he was the same as today. But it was difficult for Guillén to read his poems, which were the poems of the people, because that was the first period, the period of prejudices. Nobody ever stopped to think that for years and years, with incorruptible dedication, the poet Guillén had put all his extraordinary artistic gifts at the service of the people and at the service of the cause he believed in. The people saw in him not the glory of Cuba, but the representative of a political party that was taboo. But all that is behind us. We have already learned that we cannot have divisions based on opinions about certain internal structures in our country, if we have a common enemy and if we are trying to reach a common goal.

We all know that we have definitively become convinced that there is a common enemy. We know that everyone looks around to see if someone will hear him, if someone is listening from some embassy who will transmit their opinion, before clearly stating an opinion against the monopolies, before saying clearly: "Our enemy, and the enemy of all Latin America, is the monopolistic government of the United States of America."

If everybody already knows that this is the enemy, and if our starting point is knowing that whoever struggles against that enemy has something in common with us, then comes the second part. What are our goals here in Cuba? What do we want? Do we want the people's happiness or not? Are we struggling for Cuba's absolute economic liberation or not? Are we or are we not struggling to be a free country among free countries, without belonging to any military bloc, without having to consult any embassy of any great power on earth about any domestic or foreign decision we make? Are we thinking of redistributing the wealth of those who have too much, to give to those who have nothing? Are we thinking here of making work a creative task, a dynamic daily source of all our happiness? If so, then we already have goals to which we referred. And everyone who shares those goals is our friend. If that person also has other ideas, if they belong to one or another [political] organization, those are discussions of lesser importance.

At times of great danger, at times of great tensions and great creativity, what counts are the great enemy and the great goals. If we agree, if we all already know where we are going, then whatever happens, we must begin our work.

I was telling you that to be a revolutionary requires having a revolution. We already have [a revolution]. And a revolutionary must also know the people with whom they work. I think we still don't know one another well. I think we still have to travel a while along that road. If someone asks me how to go about getting to know the people, in addition to going into the interior [of the country], learning about cooperatives, living in cooperatives (and not everybody can do that, and there are many places where the presence of a medical doctor is very important) ... in those cases, I will tell you that one of the Cuban people's greatest expressions of solidarity is the revolutionary militias, militias that now give doctors a new function and prepare them for what was at least until recently a sad and almost fatal reality in Cuba: that is, that we were going to be prey — or if not prey at least victims — of a large-scale armed attack.

As a revolutionary militia member, the doctor should be warned to always be a doctor. They should not commit the error we made in the Sierra — or perhaps it was not an error, but all the doctor compañeros of that period know it — that it appeared dishonorable for us to be at the side of a wounded or ill person, and we sought any means possible to grab a rifle and show on the battlefield what should be done.

Now conditions are different. The new armies being formed to defend the country should be armies that use different methods, as part of which the doctor will have an enormous importance. They should continue being doctors, which is one of the most beautiful and most important tasks of war.

And not just doctors, but also nurses, laboratory technicians, all those who dedicate themselves to this humane profession.

But all of us — even knowing that the danger is latent and even while preparing to repel the aggression that still hangs over us — should stop thinking about that. Because if we center our efforts on war preparations, we cannot build what we want, we cannot devote ourselves to creative work.

All work, all capital that is invested in preparing for military action, is labor lost, money lost. Unfortunately, it has to be done, because there are others preparing. But the money I am most saddened to see leave the National Bank coffers — and I say this with all honesty and pride as a soldier — is the money to pay for some weapon of destruction.

The militias have a function in peacetime, however. The militias should be, in populated areas, the arm that unifies and gets to know the people. They should practice real solidarity, as the compañeros have told me is being done in the medical militias. They should immediately set out to resolve the problems of the impoverished throughout Cuba at all times of danger. But they are also an opportunity to get to know one another, an opportunity to live alongside people of all Cuba's social classes, made equal and made brothers by a common uniform.

If we achieve this, medical workers — and allow me to use again a term I had forgotten some time ago — if we all use that new weapon of solidarity, if we know the goals, if we know the enemy, and if we know the direction in which we have to travel, then the only thing left for us is to know the daily stretch of the road and to take it. Nobody can point out that stretch; that stretch is the personal road of each individual; it is what he or she will do every day, what a person will gain from their individual experience, and what they will give of themselves in practicing their profession, dedicated to the people's well-being.

If we already possess all the elements with which to march toward the future, let us recall that phrase of Martí, which at this moment I am not putting into practice, but which we must constantly put into practice: "The best form of saying is doing." And let us then march toward the future of Cuba.

TO UNIVERSITY STUDENTS

Speech commemorating the execution of Cuban medical students in November 1871.[17] University of Havana, November 27, 1961.

Dear compañeros:

We gather today on this stairway of struggle and remembrance — which is a symbol of the university — imbued with the new spirit of Cuban youth and with the old spirit of determination of this people, to observe a minute of remembrance for the martyrs sacrificed 90 years ago in Havana.

It has been so long since then that the image of those almost child martyrs has faded. Their memory has remained only as a symbol of colonial brutality. However, they should be remembered so that the people are always aware of what awaits them if due to some moment of hesitation, some unimaginable catastrophe, the colonial or imperialist power should return to govern Cuba.

Back then, it had already been three years since the struggle for freedom had begun. The people already knew the thousand times glorious names of Antonio Maceo and Máximo Gómez. Already back then, [José] Martí had preceded the young students on the path to imprisonment. The insurrection was advancing everywhere and the people of Cuba were fiercely fighting for their freedom.

---

[17]   On November 27, 1871, the Spanish colonial authorities executed eight medical students and sentenced dozens more to jail terms for the alleged desecration of the tomb of a Spanish loyalist.

The Volunteers, who were the first version of Masferrer's perhaps perfected and enlarged "Tigers,"[18] were the masters of Havana and owned all the strongholds that protected the colonial power. And in those times, they needed to be ruthless in the city; they had to demonstrate the power of annihilation that the Spanish colony possessed.

And so those "brave" Volunteers, who murdered children and hunted and killed blacks like wild beasts, sought out students — all of them Cubans, many of them sons of Spaniards — to demonstrate their hatred against everything that this country was.

The whole thing started when a teacher missed his classes and some of the students started to fool around on a cart that carried corpses to the morgue. Ever since the veil of religion was lifted and students began to work directly with human corpses such incidents have occurred. Young people no longer bow down before death and instead they play around with it. It is true that this is disrespectful, but all of you who have started a medical degree know that this is the case.

Apparently, in passing, one of the students plucked a flower from the cemetery. Those were the crimes committed three or four days before November 27 of that year.

On the 26th, a Spanish captain appeared and, in the presence of the teacher, took all his students prisoner. All but one exception whose name was Smith and who was American, because even at that time the United States ruled in territories populated by "inferior" people. Later, another student was freed because he was a Spaniard and a Volunteer. All the others were sent to the "cage," as the prison or dungeon was called.

That horrific legal farce was perpetrated in just a day, and the students were convicted twice. The first time, they were sentenced for desecrating a tomb, that of an "illustrious Volunteer fighter against the insurrection," but

---

18   Rolando Arcadio Masferrer Rojas was a Cuban lawyer, congressman and newspaper publisher who founded "Los Tigres de Masferrer" (Masferrer's Tigers), a paramilitary organization set up to protect dictator Fulgencio Batista. The Spanish Volunteer Corps in Cuba were considered the private militia of the Spanish colonial elite. Made up mostly of wealthy merchants and landowners, Spaniards from the metropolis known as "peninsulares," but also including their employees and some Cubans.

that was also a false accusation. On this charge, the penal code of the time condemned them to a few days in jail and a hefty fine.

Despite everything, the first court sentenced the students to that minor punishment, but the Volunteers — that is, the Tigers — demanded more. They mutinied; the beasts rioted calling for human blood.

And it was not only the blood of those executed students that was spilt in those days. Treated as an insignificant incident because it was of no importance to anyone, and even today still overlooked, the records include the discovery of five corpses of blacks killed with bayonets and bullets. But the fact that there was already strength in the people, that it was no longer possible to kill with impunity, is shown by the number of wounded Spanish scoundrels during that period.

The Volunteers demanded more and a new trial was held. Five students were condemned to death in that retrial. First, the student who had picked the flower and who confessed to it; plus four more who had climbed into the corpse cart. But a secret pact made was for eight, so three more students were drawn by lot to reach a total of eight.

I am going to read you a paragraph from a pamphlet that [José] Martí's great friend, Valdés Domínguez, who received six years in prison in that same trial, wrote later:

> See now how the Council determined those who were to be sentenced. In the first place, eight were to be executed. Alonso Álvarez de la Campa was the first to be sentenced: he had picked a flower in the cemetery, he had confessed so; Anacleto Bermúdez, José de Marcos Medina, Ángel Laborde and Pascual Rodríguez followed Álvarez de la Campa in the judges' verdict: they had played with the cart, they had stated so and they had confirmed their statement.
>
> But they were lacking another three. Lots were drawn and fate saw that dreadful accusation fall to the names of Carlos Augusto de la Torre, Carlos Verdugo and Eladio González. The name of Carlos Verdugo was drawn by chance, and the Council knew not only that he had not been in San Dionisio on the 23rd — which was the day of the incident with the carts at the cemetery — because Verdugo and all the other statements had said so, but that he had arrived from Matanzas just a few minutes before they were apprehended on the 25th.

Can anyone still dare to claim that the Council was legal? I hope never to have all the nerve necessary for such a claim. There were still 35 of us left, there was little discussion to determine our sentences; 12 of us were sentenced to six years' imprisonment, 19 to four years, and the remaining four — two Spaniards and two who were too young — to six months in minor confinement.

This was the ultimate result of the trial in which the blood of Cubans was demanded. These eight students represented the sacrifice of Cuban blood to demonstrate Spanish power; the power of the Spanish metropolis, the power of the colonists, the power of the superior race over the aboriginal races or those less pure because of their racial mixture or perhaps because of the climate.

And those young people were not guilty of anything. They can't exactly be called heroes, but rather martyrs. They were well-to-do students, because at that time students had to be from affluent families; their parents were Spanish. Álvarez de la Campa's father had been a Volunteer and until a few days before he had served in the ranks of the army, fighting against the rebellion that was gaining strength every day. His only crime was that of being Cuban.

It is true that the seed of rebellion was beginning to sprout at the university; it is true that Martí had been imprisoned for holding the ideas that would later see him lead our country in its final struggle against the enemies and take him to Dos Ríos. But there was no organized resistance in Havana, not like the resistance of the interior, of the peasants, of the rebel forces that were in the mountains and plains fighting against the Spaniards.

Were they right or wrong from their point of view to do so? I believe that according to their way of thinking, according to their reasoning as beasts accustomed to despising human life, they were right; they had to nip what was happening in the bud. Their target was wrong but if they had killed Martí, for example, what enormous damage would have been done to the revolution in later years! And nobody would have known it.

Perhaps they shot a Martí in the making there, a patriot. In any case, they annihilated "bandits' pups," and they had their reasons, because the people who were fighting against the Spanish regime at that time were very young. They were right because 15-year-old children, when a revolution is underway, are not children, they are soldiers of the homeland!

They were right, because the leader of the Rebel Youth, compañero Commander Joel Iglesias, was only 15 years old when he joined our Rebel Army a few days before the Battle of Uvero. And because 15 is an age when a person already knows what they would give their life for and is not afraid to lose it, an age when one holds an ideal in one's heart that leads a person to sacrifice themselves. That is why the Spaniards had their reasons; that is why Weyler[19] and all those who tried to annihilate the revolution were right. They sought to destroy the revolution not by killing the individual fighter, but by annihilating it among the entire population.

That is why they are right every time they unleash a brutal attack against the people, whether it be here during Spanish rule or whether it be here in the Batista period. Whether it be the Nazi hordes; whether it be colonialism of any kind, such as imperialism in Puerto Rico. They always have their reasons for trying to annihilate the people; but the people also have powerful motives. The people learn with the blows they suffer because imperialism is a great teacher at heart, and the people gradually learn to defend themselves. They become tougher, more resilient, more determined. They learn that neither the henchman's tank nor the executioner's gun are so formidable, and that the executioners are cowards when faced with people armed and ready to defend themselves.

The people learn to kill too, and one day they learn to do it so much and so well that they take power! That day came in Cuba, in an escalation of popular struggles that were born even before the November 27 [1871] that we commemorate today, that were born even before the War of 1868. With the same spirit of freedom that was present in our people when the black runaways or the indigenous people of Hatuey's era went deep into the mountains and preferred to die than live as slaves.

Thus, for years and years, the people gradually learned the difficult profession of being their own liberators. They had almost fully learned by the

---

[19]   Spanish General Valeriano Weyler y Nicolau was named governor of Cuba in 1896. In order to suppress the growing rebellion against Spanish rule, he enforced the reconcentrado policy, which saw the rural population put in concentration camps, leading to the deaths of hundreds of thousands from starvation and disease.

end of the 30 Years' War, but US imperialism intervened; they did not want the lesson to be fully learned and for 50 years all kinds of abuses were once again committed in the Republic. Today we have taken power, and it is good to recall the reason behind each of the historical events of the past. History is a great teacher. It is good to know that our present cannot become a return to the past, because it would be a terrible thing for all of us and for all the generations to follow.

We should analyze whenever possible what the past has meant for the people, and it is advisable that every time we are faced with any kind of momentary difficulty we take a look at the past and compare not the distant past, like the time of the savage execution of those eight students, but the past of today, the one you all as young people and children are familiar with: the past that ended on December 31, 1958. And let us not compare it with the present of today, with this present that we live every day, with this future that we are building with our efforts and to which you are preparing to give the final push when you have finished your degrees and have entered whatever branch of production or culture as specialists of all kinds.

All of you, the compañeros with scholarships, would do well to think about what you could have expected before the revolution. And the people, everyone, should think about what there was before every time a difficulty arises. Every time there is a "long line," every time a product is lacking — because there will be shortages and they will continue — in spite of all our efforts. Every time something goes wrong — because things will continue to go wrong despite our good intentions — we should always think of how it was in the past.

And it is helpful to always think that any difficulty that we do not know how to overcome, any small obstacle that sparks our irritation, is just a very small breach of our united front. It is worth thinking that even when that insignificant breach does not offer the slightest danger, if the difficulties mount, the gap will widen and the enemy will be able to penetrate. And it is worth remembering that to build our future we must always be united, that to strike the enemy we must strike all together, with the entire force of our people, and thus defeat him as many times as he raises his head.

But we should also remember what our duties are today. And you, compañeros, today have only one duty: the duty to study. With that duty you are repaying all the debts that you may incur to society; to this present society and to all the heroes who sacrificed themselves to make this present society possible. You are paying the debt owed by all of us to those poor students who went to their deaths without knowing why; to the great heroes who forged our nationality over 30 years of unceasing struggle; to the student heroes of this present era, from [Julio Antonio] Mella and [Rafael] Trejo to [José Antonio] Echeverría, Frank País, and the multitude of young people who gave their lives in the final years of the struggle. They did so to honor this stairway, to honor this and all Cuban universities, and to make it possible, precisely as they do today, to open their doors to everyone. To the peasant and the worker, to the white or the black student, without discrimination. To anyone who wants to study in order to better themselves, not in order to become rich with their new knowledge, but to put it at the service of society. To settle that small debt that each one of us has to the society that raises us, that dresses us and that educates us.

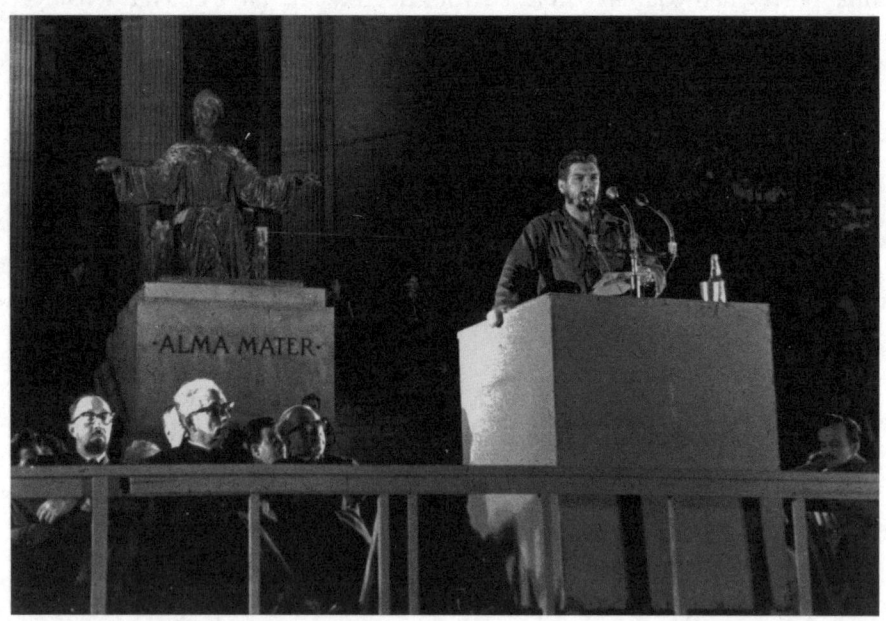

Che speaking on the steps of the University of Havana, November 27, 1961

That is the only duty. And in this way, by studying more each day, incre-asingly bettering yourselves, you honor all the compañeros who may still fall in the struggle. By also considering in every moment of weakness that the factories and the schools, the art workshops, the universities are waiting for you. That all of Cuba is waiting for you and that you cannot waste a minute, because we are all moving toward the future, and the future needs techno-logy, it needs culture, it needs high revolutionary consciousness.

On one of the many occasions on which José Martí referred to this sad episode of the assassination of the students, he wrote some words that could serve as the perfect close to this new day of remembrance, on the 90th anni-versary of the execution of our compañeros. Martí said something very simple and very beautiful, like all the things he said:

> We love our brothers who died more each day. We do not wish that they rest in peace, because they live on in the sublime restlessness of glory. Today we shed one more tear in their memory, and we are inspired to mourn them for their vigor and courage. Weep with us all those who feel, suffer with us all those who love! Fall to your knees upon the earth, trem-ble with remorse, groan with dread, all those who on that terrible day hel-ped to kill!

And that is what we can say today: that we do not wish that they rest in peace, that we also wish that they may live by our side in the present and that they may merge with this new Cuba, which advances toward the future without fear of anyone or anything, ready to work harder every day, ready to perfect itself every day. Ready to be increasingly deserving of what we are today for the entire Americas: the highest beacon, the greatest hope, the most perfect example!

INTERNATIONAL
MISSIONS

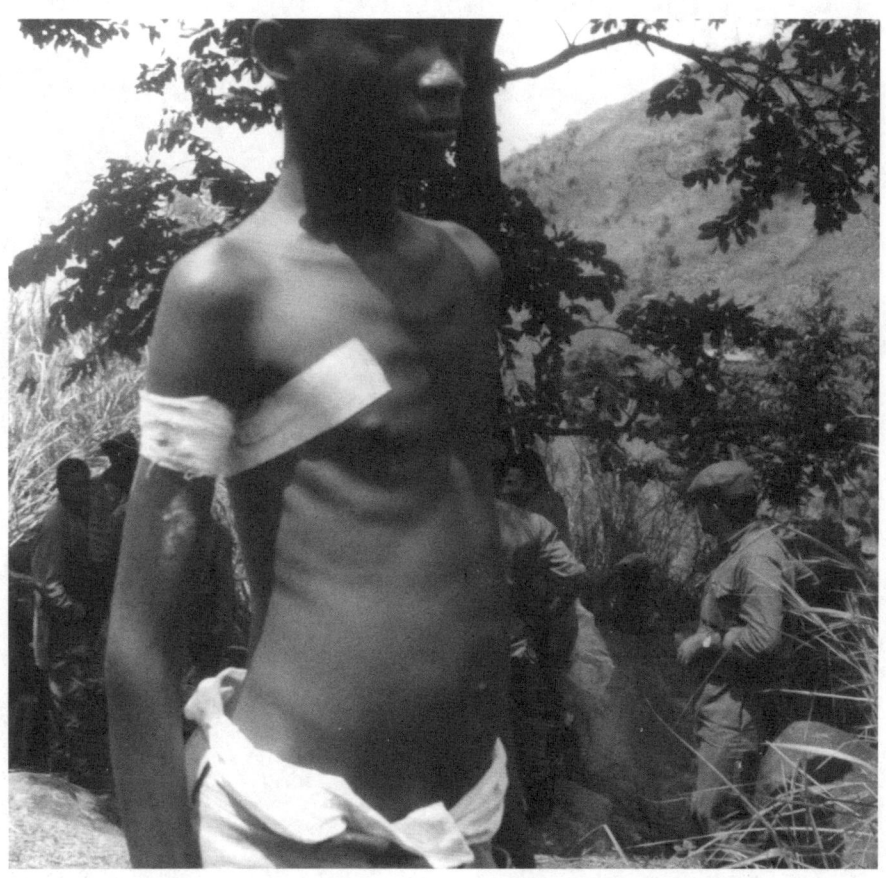

Visiting a camp for the wounded in the Congo.

THE CONGO

Excerpts from *Che's Congo Diary: Episodes of the Revolutionary War in the Congo.*

Our country, the sole socialist bastion on the doorstep of Yankee imperialism, sends its soldiers to fight and die in a foreign land, on a distant continent, and publicly assumes full responsibility for its actions. In this challenge, in this clear position on the great modern-day issue of waging a relentless struggle against Yankee imperialism, lies the heroic significance of our participation in the struggle of the Congo. *("Preface: An Initial Warning.")*

[...]

Lieutenant-Colonel Lambert explained with a friendly, cheerful spirit that airplanes had no importance for them because they had *dawa*, a medicine that makes a person invulnerable to bullets.

"I've been hit a number of times, but the bullets simply fell to the ground." He said this with a smile on his face, and I felt obliged to respond to the joke, which I saw as a sign of how little importance they attached to the enemy's weapons. But I soon realized it was meant seriously, that the magical protection of *dawa* was one of the great weapons of triumph of the Congolese army.

This *dawa* did a lot of damage to military preparedness. It operates according to the following principle: A liquid in which herbal substances and other magical ingredients have been dissolved is thrown over the combatant, and certain occult markers — nearly always including a coal mark on the forehead — are administered to him. This protects him against all kinds of weapons (although the enemy too relies upon magic), but he must not touch anything not belonging to him, touch a woman or feel fear, or the protection will be ineffective. The reason for any failure was very simple: a dead man is one who became fearful, stole or slept with a woman; and anyone wounded is someone who succumbed to fear. As fear accompanies war, wounds were quite naturally attributed to fear — that is, to a lack of faith. And as the dead cannot speak, all three transgressions can be readily ascribed to them.

This belief is so strong that no one goes into battle without having the *dawa* performed on them. I was constantly afraid that this superstition would rebound against us, and that we would be blamed for any military disaster involving a lot of casualties. I tried several times to discuss the *dawa* with those in leadership positions in an effort to win people away from it — but this was impossible. The *dawa* is treated as an article of faith. Even the most politically developed argued that it is a natural, material force and that they, as dialectical materialists, recognized the power of the *dawa*, whose secrets lie with jungle medicine men.

[...]

In my capacity as a doctor (an epidemiologist — which, if this illustrious branch of the Aesculapian fauna forgives me for saying so, entitled me to know nothing about medicine), I worked for a few days with Kumi at the clinic and noticed several alarming facts: the first being the high number of cases of venereal disease, often due to infection picked up in Kigoma. What concerned me at the time was not the state of health of the general population and the prostitutes of Kigoma, in particular, but the fact that the frequent trips across the lake meant many of our combatants could become infected. Other questions also arose. Who paid those women? Where did the money come from? How were the revolution's funds being spent?

From the first few days of our stay, we also had the opportunity to see some cases of alcohol poisoning caused by the famous *pombe*. This is a spirit distilled from fermented corn and cassava flour, which is not so high in alcohol content but the distilled liquor has terrible effects. Presumably these arise not so much from the concentration of the alcohol itself as from the amount of impurities contained in the liquor due to the rudimentary method of its production. There were days when the camp was awash with *pombe*, leaving behind a trail of brawling, drunkenness, indiscipline, etc.

Peasants from the surrounding area began to visit the clinic after hearing on "Radio Bemba" [word of mouth] that there were doctors in the area. Our supply of medicines was poor, but a Soviet medical consignment came to our aid. It had not been selected with a civilian population in mind, but naturally to meet the needs of an army in the field — and even then, it did not contain an adequate range of medicines.

[...]

Our morale remained high although complaints were starting to be heard among the compañeros as they watched the days pass unproductively. Also hovering over us was the specter of malaria and the other tropical fevers that struck nearly everyone in one form or another; these often responded to malaria drugs, but left behind troublesome aftereffects, such as general debility or lack of appetite, which added to the incipient pessimism creeping into the troop's morale.

As the days went by, the picture of organizational chaos became more evident. I myself took part in the distribution of Soviet medical supplies and this resembled a gypsy marketplace; each representative of the armed groups produced figures, and cited facts and reasons why he should have access to a greater amount of medicine. There were several conflicts as I tried to stop some medicine or special equipment being unnecessarily carried off to the front lines, but everyone wanted everything. They started to claim incredible numbers of combatants in their group: one declared 4,000, another 2,000, etc. These were inventions ...

[...]

During these days, the various fronts were almost completely passive and if people had gunshot wounds to be attended, these were the result of accidents. Since hardly anyone had the faintest idea about firearms, they tended to go off when they were played with or treated carelessly.

[...]

Kabila sent word that I should be very circumspect about my identity and so I remained incognito as I acted in my apparent role as doctor and translator.

We agreed with Mitoudidi that the move to Upper Base would take place the next day. This happened, but we left behind Moja, Nane and Tano, who had come down with fever, and the doctor Kumi to take care of the hospital. I was sent to the base as doctor and translator. There were scarcely 20 Congolese there, looking bored, lonely and uncomfortable. The struggle began to break this inertia; we started with classes in Swahili, given by the political commissar at the base, and in French, assigned to another compañero. We also started building shelters as protection against the freezing temperatures. We were at 1,700 meters above sea level and 1,000 meters above the level of the lake, in an area where trade winds from the Indian Ocean condense causing continuous rainfall. We immediately commenced the task of building shelters, and we soon had blazing fires to ward off the nocturnal cold. *("First Impressions.")*

[...]

In my first few days at the Upper Base, I paid tribute to the climate of the Congo by coming down with a very high, though short-lived, fever. Our doctor, Kumi, came up from the Lake [Base] to visit me, but I sent him back as he was needed in the clinic and I was already feeling better. On the third or fourth day they brought in a man wounded in some skirmish at Front de Force; he had not received medical attention for six days, so his arm that had been fractured by a bullet was now suppurating profusely. I had to get up to attend to him in a cold drizzle, and this may have caused my relapse with a very high fever and delirium, bringing Kumi up to the base for a second time. It was like climbing Mount Everest for him, and according to eyewitnesses — because I was in no state to appreciate the fact — his condition after the long, steep ascent appeared worse than that of the patient he had come to attend. *("The First Month.")*

[...]

To protect myself from the rigors of the climate, I lay on a hide very close to the fire. I slept well, but immediately fell prey to one of the local fiends, the *birulo*, a louse that lives mainly in clothing and roams freely all over this region of relatively temperate climate and zero hygiene.

[...]

The peasants were extremely friendly toward us, and I felt very much in their debt so that I returned to my old profession as a doctor, reduced under the circumstances to the bare minimum of penicillin injections against gonorrhea, the local disease, and tablets against malaria. *("Scattering Seeds.")*

[...]

In accordance with our principles, we launched the beginnings of social programs. Dr. Hindi, who had arrived from the base, began seeing the local peasants and established a schedule of visits to the mountain villages. I distributed legume seeds brought from the lake, so that some vegetables could be sown and cultivated and later provided to us. We managed to create a different, more communicative atmosphere. Like peasants anywhere in the world, they were responsive to any human interest shown to them; they were grateful and very cooperative. *("Attempting 'Pursuit'.")*

[…]

We spoke for a long time with the peasants; as we had no medicines with us, I asked Makungu to send a doctor to attend to some sick people and I promised that a doctor would drop by every fortnight on scheduled rounds.

[…]

Inside the vehicle was an individual with all the signs of alcohol poisoning, including dreadful vomiting. I found out the next day that he had died in Fizi's hospital — or receptacle would be a better word, because it had no doctors or medical assistance of any kind.

[…]

Before we left, they took me around Fizi and I had an opportunity to examine a wounded man from Kasengo. The bullet had gone through muscle, and the untreated wound had become infected and was emitting a nauseating smell (he had spent a fortnight like this). I recommended that he should be sent without delay to Kibamba for treatment by the doctors there, and suggested we could take advantage of our own trip to take him right away as far as Baraka. They considered it was more important to put a large escort on the truck and to leave the wounded man in Fizi; I heard no more about him, but I imagine he didn't do so well. *("Taking the Pulse.")*

[…]

We held a meeting with the chairman of one of the nearby villages. Each small village has its *kapita* or chief, and the large ones — or a group of hamlets — have a chairman. Our man spoke French and was quite smart. In the course of a long conversation, I presented our requests: we needed some people to go to the Lake [Base] and bring back food and other supplies; the peasants would provide us with cassava, some vegetables and raw tobacco. What we could offer was some of the food and other items brought up from the Lake [Base], payment for the food they provided, free medical care and medicines within our means, and vegetable seeds (whose produce we would share). The chairman noted everything down and held a meeting with his compañeros; after two or three days he ceremoniously brought me a signed typewritten reply with a multiple of stamps that stated he would find men to send to the Lake [Base], that they would guarantee us food and try to find tobacco, but that he could not accept payment because it was revolutionary norm that the peasants were to feed and support the army and they would keep this norm.

[...]

Machado and I agreed that it was impossible to have 50 doctors here, unless we organized them as a guerrilla unit. He also agreed with me about the genuinely alarming aspects of the situation as he had witnessed all the depravity at the fronts and had developed a feel for the spirit of this revolution.

I had hoped that some compañeros, such as the local minister of public health, might help to create a little order, especially because he came from the Fizi area and had some authority. But he proved to be a nobody. He remained there until the end, except for a brief time when he left on account of something to do with his work, but he kept completely detached from Massengo (I can't say which of them was to blame) and even more detached from reality. Of course, he could not occupy himself with public health; he had only the Cuban doctors, and the few medicines that arrived were for the fronts or for some primary care in the areas where our forces were based. We had once spoken with Massengo of the need to concern ourselves more with Fizi, to impose authority on the general and pay him some attention (as far as doctors and the radio were concerned, for example), but that was now history as Fizi had become enemy territory. *("A Battle against Time.")*

[...]

The effects of the climate were still being felt, as gastroenteritis was added to the endemic malaria. Until the rigors of the task got the better of my scientific spirit, I noted in my field diary my own statistics: I had the shits more than 30 times in 24 hours. Only the bush knows how many more there were after that. Many compañeros suffered from the same malady; it didn't last long and it responded to strong antibiotics, but it contributed to undermining an already fragile morale. *("Various Escapes.")*

[...]

While Bahasa was being treated, we took the sides of the hill because we were still in a valley. The bullet had completely shattered his humerus and a rib and penetrated his lung. The wound reminded me of a compañero I had tended to years before in Cuba, who had died within a few hours. Bahasa was stronger, his stronger bones had slowed the bullet down, and it didn't seem to have reached his mediastinum. But he was clearly in great pain. A splint was applied as best we could, and we began a most tiring ascent through steep hills slippery from the rain. The very heavy load was carried by exhausted men, who did not get full cooperation from their Congolese compañeros.

[...]

Bahasa seemed to improve. He spoke and felt a little less pain (although he was still very agitated), and was able to drink some chicken broth. Reassured by his condition, I took a photo in which his large, habitually bulging eyes expressed an anxiety that we had not known how to allay.

At dawn on October 26, the nurse came to tell me that Bahasa had had a crisis, ripped off his bandages and died, apparently of an acute haematothorax. Later that morning we had to carry out the sad and solemn ritual of digging a grave and burying Compañero Bahasa, the sixth man we had lost and the first whose body could be given the appropriate honors. It was a mute and powerful accusation against my stupidity and lack of foresight, as had been Bahasa's brave conduct from the moment he was wounded. *("Disaster.")*

[...]

An unfortunate incident helped to ensure the peasants' quick and enthusiastic response to our appeal. At the Lubondja barrier, a group of Congolese decided to set up some grenade-traps for greenhorns but did not inform their compañeros; another group of Congolese passed by and fell into the trap designed for the enemy. Three slightly wounded men came in for treatment, plus a fourth with a more serious stomach perforation that they attributed to a mortar round fired by the advancing enemy. Those slightly wounded were soon treated, but the other man had to have a delicate intestinal operation in the open air, under very difficult conditions, with a constant threat from aircraft flying over the area. In spite of everything, the operation was a success and raised the respect for Compañero Morogoro, the surgeon, and allowed us to insist on the rapid completion of the hospital, at a quiet and peaceful spot where such tasks could be carried out in proper safety.

That same evening, another wounded man came in with a double perforation. What had happened? The whole group had fled when they heard the explosion; the slightly wounded man and the man with the stomach wound, who was able to help himself, also took to their heels and were later picked up by their compañeros. But no one stayed behind, possibly because his condition was too serious for him to be moved, or perhaps simply because he was terrified. With night approaching, it was clear that the guardsmen were not advancing and some of the Congolese resolved to go back closer and retrieve the weapons they had thrown away in their flight. It was then that they came across the wounded compañero and brought him to the hospital during the night. We had no lamps or proper lighting, nor adequate drugs, and so an even more difficult operation than the previous one had to be performed by the light of just a couple of lanterns on a man in a terrible physical state. At dawn, when the four perforations had finally been treated, the patient died. All these efforts, as well as our care for a woman wounded in a strange struggle with a buffalo (which was eventually killed with spears), did a lot to lift the peasants' regard for us and to help us form a nucleus capable of withstanding the malignant influence of the commanders. ("*The Whirlwind.*")

BOLIVIA

Excerpts from *Che's The Bolivian Diary.*

1967: January

Alejandro is showing signs of malaria. (*January 16*)

Miguel came down with a high fever and has all the symptoms of malaria. I felt like I was coming down with something, but nothing developed. (*January 19*)

Miguel still has a high fever. (*January 20*).

Miguel is getting better, but Carlos now has a high fever.

A tuberculin test was administered today. (*January 22*)

[...] Carlos still is running a fever, typical of malaria. (*January 23*)

1967: February

El Médico [Moro] treated the children who had worms and a mare had kicked one of them; then we headed off. (*February 10*)

Inti is unwell; he has gas pains for the second time in a week. (*February 21*)

We set out at noon, with the sun strong enough to split rocks, and a little later, when we reached the crest of the highest hill, I felt faint; from then on, I kept going from sheer determination. The highest point in this area is 1,420 meters, a summit that overlooks a wide area that includes the Río Grande, the mouth of the Ñacahuazú, and part of the Rosita. (*February 23*)

1967: March

The men's morale is low; Miguel has swollen feet and several others have a similar condition. (*March 15*)

We decided to eat the horse because swollen feet is now an alarming problem. Miguel, Inti, Urbano, and Alejandro all have various symptoms; I am extremely weak.

[...]

Message 32 has been completely decoded, reporting the arrival of a Bolivian who will join us, with another load of Glucantine, an antiparasitic medication for leishmania. Up to now we have had no cases. (*March 16*)

1967: April

The first reports soon arrived, with unfortunate news. Rubio [Jesús Suárez Gayol] had been mortally wounded. His body was carried to our camp; he had been shot in the head. (*April 10*)

The vanguard set out at 6:15 and we left at 7:15, walking at a good pace to the Iquira River, but Tania and Alejandro fell behind. When their temperatures were taken, Tania's was over 39 degrees and Alejandro's was about 38. Moreover, the delay prevented us from progressing as we had planned. We left the two of them, along with Negro and Serapio, a kilometer up the Iquira and we proceed to occupy the hamlet [...]. (*April 16*)

Moisés must stay with the group of stragglers because of an acute gallbladder attack. (*April 17*)

When the shooting was over, I sent Urbano to order a retreat, but he came back with the news that Rolando was wounded. Shortly, they brought him back, but he was already dying; he died as we began to give him plasma. A bullet had split his femur and all the surrounding nerves and vessels; he bled to death before we could do anything. (*April 25*)

On another level, we are totally cut off; illness has undermined the health of some compañeros, obliging us to divide our forces, which has greatly reduced our effectiveness; we have still not made contact with Joaquín [...] (*Summary of the month*)

1967: May

The only food we have left is lard; I felt faint and had to sleep two hours to be able to continue at even this slow and hesitant pace; in general, the march has been that way. We ate soup made from the lard at the first water hole. The troops are sick and now many have edema. (*May 9*)

A day of burps, farts, vomiting, and diarrhea — a real concert from our organs. We remained completely immobile trying to digest the pig. We have two cans of water. I was feeling very bad until I vomited and then felt better. (*May 13*)

Just as we started out, I came down with intense abdominal pain, with vomiting and diarrhea. I got it under control with Demerol, but lost consciousness and had to be carried in a hammock. When I awoke I felt much better, but I was covered in shit like a newborn baby. I borrowed a pair of pants, but without water, the stench could be smelled for a league away. We spent the whole day there, with me dozing. (*May 16*)

Raúl has an abscess on his knee and cannot walk because of the intense pain; he was given a strong antibiotic and tomorrow it will have to be lanced. We walked some 15 kilometers (*May 17*)

Raúl's abscess was lanced and 50cc of purulent liquid was drained; he was given a general treatment to fight infection; he can barely take a step. I performed my first tooth extraction for this guerrilla campaign; the fortunate victim: Camba — everything went well. (*May 18*)

Raúl is slowly improving; his abscess was lanced again and another 40cc of purulent liquid was drained. He no longer has a fever, but he is in pain and can barely walk; he is my current concern. (*May 21*)

1967: June

After two days of profuse dental extractions, which made me famous as "Fernando Sacamuelas" [Tooth-puller] alias Chaco, I closed my clinic and we set off in the afternoon, walking just over an hour. (*June 21*)

Asthma is becoming a serious problem for me and there is very little medicine left. (*June 23*)

My asthma is worsening. (*June 24*)

The withdrawal was delayed and we got news of two wounded: Pombo in his leg and Tuma in his abdomen. We carried them quickly to the house to operate on them the best we could. Pombo's wound is superficial and will just cause headaches because of his lack of mobility. Tuma's wound destroyed his liver and produced intestinal perforations; he died during the operation. With his death, I have lost an inseparable compañero of recent years, one whose loyalty was unwavering and whose absence I feel now almost as if he were my own son. (*June 26*)

1967: July

Pombo's leg is not improving fast enough, probably due to the interminable trips on horseback, but there are no complications, nor fear of any at this point. (*July 2*)

My asthma continues to wage war. (*July 3*)

Asthma punished me severely and for the first time would not let me sleep at all. (*July 4*)

I injected myself several times so I could continue, finally, using an eyewash solution containing 1/900 adrenaline. If Paulino has not accomplished his mission, we will have to return to Ñacahuazú to retrieve my asthma medication. (*July 8*)

My asthma hit me hard and those measly few sedatives are just about gone. (*July 27*)

Things happened like this: Ricardo and Aniceto were imprudently crossing the clearing when Ricardo was wounded. Antonio organized a line of fire between Arturo, Aniceto, and Pacho, and they rescued him, but then Pacho was wounded and a bullet to the mouth killed Raúl. The withdrawal was difficult, dragging the two wounded men [...].

Pacho came on horseback but Ricardo could not ride and they had to carry him in a hammock. I sent Miguel, with Pablito, Darío, Coco, and Aniceto, to occupy the mouth of the first creek to the right, while we tended the wounded. Pacho had a superficial wound that went through his buttocks and the skin of his testicles, but Ricardo was in critical condition and the last plasma had been lost in Willy's backpack. Ricardo died at 22:00 and we buried him near the river, in a well-hidden place so that the soldiers could not find him. (*July 30*).

1967: August

My asthma is hitting me very hard and I have used up my last anti-asthmatic injection; all I have left are tablets for about 10 days. (*August 2*)

Pacho is recuperating; on the other hand, I am not doing so well; I had a bad day and a bad night and I have no idea how a solution will be found in the short term. I tried an intravenous Novocain injection, to no avail. (*August 3*)

An abscess on my heel was lanced, allowing me to put weight on my foot, but it is still very painful and I am running a fever.

Pacho is fine. (*August 9*)

My foot was treated again. I am getting better, but I am not well yet. (*August 10*)

[...] Pacho is recovering at a good rate, and my asthma has been getting worse since yesterday; I am now taking three tablets a day. My foot is almost better. (*August 13*)

It was cold, but I did not have a bad night; another abscess on my same foot needs to be lanced. Pacho is back on his feet. (*August 15*)

I ate urina and it gave me a severe asthma attack in the middle of the night. El Médico is apparently still suffering from lumbago, which is affecting his general health and turning him into an invalid. (*August 20*)

I gave El Médico a local anesthetic so he could travel on the mare, although it was still painful; he seems to have improved slightly; Pacho made the trip on foot. (*August 22*)

El Médico is still in pain and is giving himself Talamonal; I am fairly well [...] (*August 24*)

The situation is becoming distressing now; the macheteros are fainting, Miguel and Darío are drinking their own urine, as is Chino, with the disastrous result of diarrhea and cramps. (*August 30*)

1967: September

A day of stomatology; I extracted teeth from Arturo and Chapaco [...] (*September 17*)

By the time we reached the settlement called Loma Larga, I had pains in my liver and was vomiting; the troops are exhausted from these unproductive hikes. (September 24)

A few moments later, Benigno arrived, wounded, followed by Aniceto and Pablito, with a foot in a bad way. Miguel, Coco, and Julio had been killed [...] (*September 26*)

Benigno is fine, but El Médico has not fully recovered. (*September 30*)

1967: October

   We took care of Benigno, whose wound was oozing a bit, and I gave El Médico an injection. As a result of the treatment, Benigno complained of pain during the night. (*October 5*)

Che's last diary entry was October 7. The next day he was captured and executed in cold blood on October 9

BY WAY OF AN EPILOGUE:
Why I became a doctor
By Dr. Aleida Guevara

I was raised on this Caribbean island of Cuba and I am the fruit of immense love. Both my parents are my greatest role models. But as my father was absent for most of my childhood, from a very young age I decided I would be a doctor, probably because he was. Of course, as time passed, my commitment to the medical profession strengthened, as I hoped to give back some of the love I had received from my people. Deciding to be a doctor was the best way I saw I could be useful to my people and others around the world.

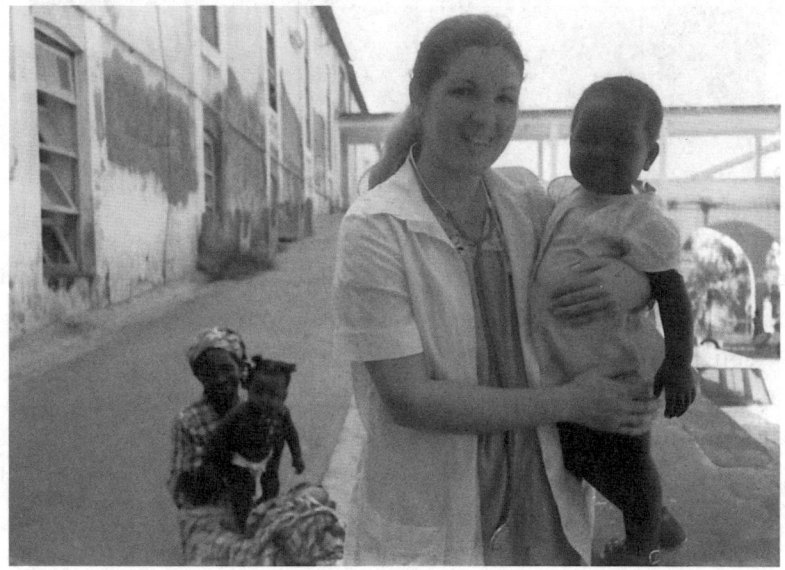

This is more or less how I came to choose my profession. What is certain is that I really enjoy what I do. I feel fulfilled when I receive the affection of my Cuban patients, although there is no doubt that my father Che's example has encouraged me to carry out my duties in other countries of the world. He used to say that solidarity was not to be practiced from afar, that solidarity meant to share the lives of people.

The Sandinista revolution triumphed in Nicaragua as I was finishing my medical degree. At the time, Cuba did not have enough doctors to send to that country, where the population was in urgent need of care. So Fidel Castro talked with medical students to see who would like to undertake their final year residency abroad. Over 400 from my course alone volunteered.

It was an unforgettable experience, and I could recount thousands of anecdotes, how much I learned there. I would say that it made us better professionals and, above all, better human beings.

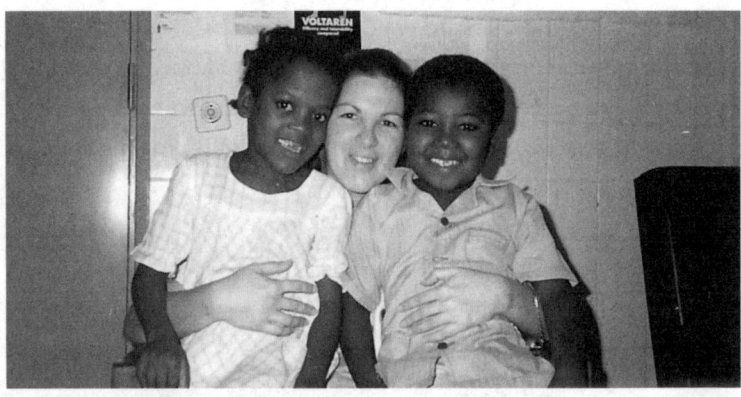

Some years later I went to Angola, in the midst of the war against Apartheid in Southern Africa. There, we young Cubans worked hard to save lives — in my case those of children — in a place far from home, motivated by the conviction that we were giving back a little of all that we owe to the immense continent of Africa. We Cubans are the fruit of that culture too.

I shed many a tear as I experienced glorious but also terribly sad moments alongside the Angolan people. My memories are full of the faces of children suffering from tuberculosis, among whom I sought comfort, love and the strength needed to face the harsh reality that struck us every day working at Luanda's María Pía hospital (later renamed the Josina Machel hospital).

It was a relentless fight against all forms of colonialism, exploitation, racial discrimination and everything representing the legacy of imperialism. I am the product of the internationalist education that the Cuban revolution instills in its children: respect for the lives of all human beings, in any part of the world.

That is why I work with the Brazilian Landless Workers' Movement. I have provided consultations in Esmeralda and Cotacachi, in Ecuador. It has also given me great pleasure to work with the Fundación Un Mundo Mejor es Posible (A Better World is Possible Foundation) and its Che Guevara Medical Brigade, made up of young graduate doctors from Cuba's Latin American School of Medicine (ELAM) and Argentines of different medical specialties, with whom we have visited places such as Gan Gan, in Patagonia; Humahuaca in Jujuy province; Dorado in Misiones province; Santo Lugares in the province of Santiago del Estero; and Valle de Traslasierras in Córdoba province.

In recent years, I have worked in municipalities of Michoacán State, Mexico, including Nueva Italia, Uruapan, Paracho and San Juan Nuevo. I always strive to do my best in fulfilling my social role as a doctor.

For me, one of the most beautiful things that has happened in my life, was when my youngest daughter announced she wanted to study medicine. This surprised me because she was a real runabout as a teenager. She was lucky not to be thrown out of school because she would never study.

Then one day she tells me: "I am going to be a doctor." She had completed all her pre-university years in an IT technical school, so I thought that if she was going to continue studying it would be something related to IT, possibly cybernetics. "What did you say?" I responded. "Do you think I can't do it?" she said. "No," I said, "but my girl, you have been studying mathematics for three years, and medicine is pure biology, so how are you going to manage?" She replied, "Don't worry, I am going to be a doctor."

Let me tell you that she is a tremendous vascular surgeon, and I'm not saying that just because she is my daughter but because her patients say so. They all speak very well of her, with much respect. When she operates on a patient, she stays with that patient until she has stabilized them, she does not leave their side — that is the mark of a doctor who respects her profession.

She is now specializing in cardiovascular surgery, because she not only wants to be able to operate the peripheral vessels, but she also wants to operate the major vessels. For that she has to do cardiovascular surgery; she is now in her fourth year of the specialty.

This is why our Che lives on and remains present among those who are convinced that solidarity is the greatest expression of kindness among peoples, and that only by practicing solidarity as we Cubans do, can we build a better world for all.

¡Hasta la Victoria Siempre!

Aleida Guevara March is a pediatrician who specializes in childhood allergies.

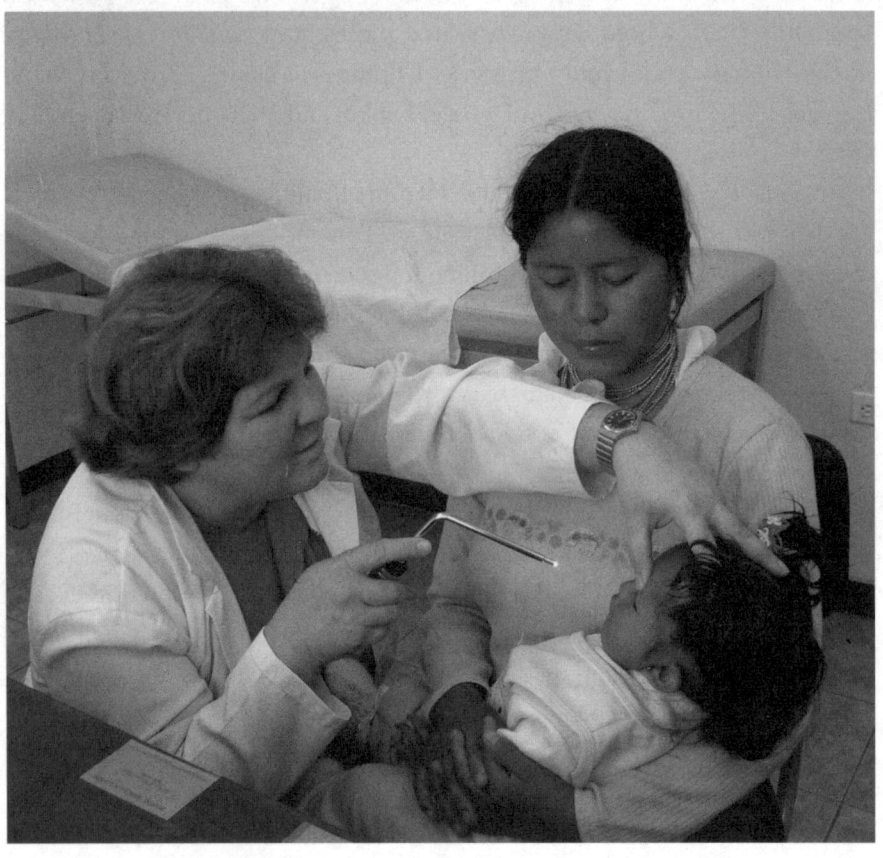

BOOKS BY ERNESTO CHE GUEVARA

The Motorcycle Diaries: Notes on a Latin American Journey.

Latin America Diaries: Otra Vez or a Second Look at Latin America.

The Awakening of Latin America: A Classic Anthology of Che Guevara's Writings on Latin America.

Reminiscences of the Cuban Revolutionary War.

Guerrilla Warfare.

The Bolivian Diary.

Congo Diary: Episodes of the Revolutionary War in the Congo.

Che: The Diaries of Ernesto Che Guevara.

Self Portrait: A Photographic and Literary Memoir.

Global Justice: Liberation and Socialism.

Che Guevara Reader: Writings on Politics and Revolution.

CHE GUEVARA PUBLISHING PROJECT

www.cheguevaralibros.com

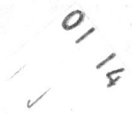